Lecture Notes in Computer Science 10530

Commenced Publication in 1973
Founding and Former Series Editors:
Gerhard Goos, Juris Hartmanis, and Jan van Leeuwen

Editorial Board

David Hutchison
Lancaster University, Lancaster, UK
Takeo Kanade
Carnegie Mellon University, Pittsburgh, PA, USA
Josef Kittler
University of Surrey, Guildford, UK
Jon M. Kleinberg
Cornell University, Ithaca, NY, USA
Friedemann Mattern
ETH Zurich, Zurich, Switzerland
John C. Mitchell
Stanford University, Stanford, CA, USA
Moni Naor
Weizmann Institute of Science, Rehovot, Israel
C. Pandu Rangan
Indian Institute of Technology, Madras, India
Bernhard Steffen
TU Dortmund University, Dortmund, Germany
Demetri Terzopoulos
University of California, Los Angeles, CA, USA
Doug Tygar
University of California, Berkeley, CA, USA
Gerhard Weikum
Max Planck Institute for Informatics, Saarbrücken, Germany

More information about this series at http://www.springer.com/series/7412

Guorong Wu · Brent C. Munsell
Yiqiang Zhan · Wenjia Bai
Gerard Sanroma · Pierrick Coupé (Eds.)

Patch-Based Techniques in Medical Imaging

Third International Workshop, Patch-MI 2017
Held in Conjunction with MICCAI 2017
Quebec City, QC, Canada, September 14, 2017
Proceedings

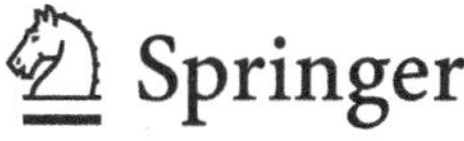

Editors
Guorong Wu
University of North Carolina at Chapel Hill
Chapel Hill, NC
USA

Brent C. Munsell
College of Charleston
Charleston, SC
USA

Yiqiang Zhan
Siemens Medical Solutions
Malvern, PA
USA

Wenjia Bai
Imperical College London
London
UK

Gerard Sanroma
Pompeu Fabra University
Barcelona
Spain

Pierrick Coupé
Bordeaux University
Talence Cedex
France

ISSN 0302-9743 ISSN 1611-3349 (electronic)
Lecture Notes in Computer Science
ISBN 978-3-319-67433-9 ISBN 978-3-319-67434-6 (eBook)
DOI 10.1007/978-3-319-67434-6

Library of Congress Control Number: 2017952846

LNCS Sublibrary: SL6 – Image Processing, Computer Vision, Pattern Recognition, and Graphics

© Springer International Publishing AG 2017
This work is subject to copyright. All rights are reserved by the Publisher, whether the whole or part of the material is concerned, specifically the rights of translation, reprinting, reuse of illustrations, recitation, broadcasting, reproduction on microfilms or in any other physical way, and transmission or information storage and retrieval, electronic adaptation, computer software, or by similar or dissimilar methodology now known or hereafter developed.
The use of general descriptive names, registered names, trademarks, service marks, etc. in this publication does not imply, even in the absence of a specific statement, that such names are exempt from the relevant protective laws and regulations and therefore free for general use.
The publisher, the authors and the editors are safe to assume that the advice and information in this book are believed to be true and accurate at the date of publication. Neither the publisher nor the authors or the editors give a warranty, express or implied, with respect to the material contained herein or for any errors or omissions that may have been made. The publisher remains neutral with regard to jurisdictional claims in published maps and institutional affiliations.

Printed on acid-free paper

This Springer imprint is published by Springer Nature
The registered company is Springer International Publishing AG
The registered company address is: Gewerbestrasse 11, 6330 Cham, Switzerland

Preface

Patch-based techniques play an increasingly important role in the medical imaging field, with various applications in image segmentation, image de-noising, image super-resolution, super-pixel/voxel-based analysis, computer-aided diagnosis, image registration, abnormality detection, and image synthesis. Dictionaries of local image patches are increasingly being used for example in the context of segmentation and computer-aided diagnosis. Patch-based dictionaries are commonly used in conjunction with pattern recognition techniques to model complex anatomies in an accurate and easy way. The patch-level representation of image content is between the global image and localized voxels. This level of representation is shown to be successful in areas such as image processing (e.g., enhancement and de-noising) as well as image feature extraction and classification (e.g., convolution kernels and convolutional neural networks).

The main aim of this workshop series is to help advance scientific research within the broad field of patch-based processing in medical imaging. It focuses on major trends and challenges in this area, and it presents work aiming to identify new cutting-edge techniques and their use in medical imaging. We hope that this workshop series will become a new platform for translating research from bench to bedside and for presenting original, high-quality papers on innovative research and development in the analysis of medical image data using patch-based techniques.

Topics of interests include but are not limited to patch-based processing dedicated to:

- Image segmentation of anatomical structures or lesions (e.g., brain segmentation, cardiac segmentation, MS lesions detection, tumor segmentation)
- Image enhancement (e.g., de-noising or super-resolution dedicated to fMRI, DWI, MRI, or CT)
- Computer-aided prognostic and diagnostic (e.g., for lung cancer, prostate cancer, breast cancer, colon cancer, brain diseases, liver cancer, acute disease, chronic disease, osteoporosis)
- Mono and multimodal image registration
- Multi-modality fusion (e.g., MRI/PET, PET/CT, projection X-ray/CT, X-ray/ultrasound) for diagnosis, image analysis, and image-guided interventions
- Mono and multi modal image synthesis (e.g., synthesis of missing a modality in a database using an external library)
- Image retrieval (e.g., context-based retrieval, lesion similarity)
- Dynamic, functional, physiologic, and anatomic imaging
- Super-pixel/voxel-based analysis in medical images
- Sparse dictionary learning and sparse coding
- Analysis of 2D, 2D+t, 3D, 3D+t, 4D, and 4D+t data.

An academic objective of the workshop is to bring together researchers in medical imaging to discuss new techniques using patch-based approaches and their use in clinical decision support and large cohort studies. Another objective is to explore new paradigms in the design of biomedical image analysis systems that exploit the latest results in patch-based processing and exemplar-based methods. MICCAI-PMI 2017 featured a single-track workshop with keynote speakers, technical paper presentations, poster sessions, and demonstrations of state-of-the-art techniques and concepts that are applied to analyzing medical images.

We received a total of 26 submissions. All papers underwent a rigorous double-blind review process by at least 2 members (mostly 3 members) of the Program Committee composed of 38 well-known experts in the field. The séléction of the papers was based on significance of results, technical merit, relevance, and clarity of presentation. Based on the reviewing scores and critiques, the 18 best papers were accepted for presentation at the workshop and chosen to be included in the present proceedings.

Authors of selected papers will be invited to submit an extended version to the PatchMI Special Issue in the *Computerized Medical Imaging and Graphics Journal.*

July 2017

G. Wu
B. Munsell
Y. Zhan
W. Bai
G. Sanroma
P. Coupé

Organization

Program Committee

Charles Kervrann	Inria Rennes - Bretagne Atlantique, France
Dinggang Shen	UNC Chapel Hill, USA
Daniel Rueckert	Imperial College, UK
Francois Rousseau	Télécom Bretagne, France
Gang Li	UNC Chapel Hill, USA
Guoyan Zheng	University of Bern, Switzerland
Islem Rekik	University of Dundee, UK
Jean-Francois Mangin	I2BM, France
Jerome Boulanger	IRISA, France
Jerry Prince	Johns Hopkins University, USA
José Vicente Manjón	ITACA Institute, Polytechnic University of Valencia, Spain
Juan Eugenio Iglesias	University College London, UK
Julia Schnabel	King's College London, UK
Junzhou Huang	University of Texas at Arlington, USA
Jussi Tohka	Universidad Carlos III de Madrid, Spain
Karim Lekadir	Universitat Pompeu Fabra, Spain
Li Shen	Indiana University, USA
Li Wang	UNC Chapel Hill, USA
Lin Yang	University of Florida, USA
Martin Styner	UNC Chapel Hill, USA
Mattias Heinrich	University of Luebeck, Germany
Mert Sabuncu	Cornell University, USA
Olivier Colliot	UPMC, France
Olivier Commowick	Inria, France
Paul Yushkevich	UPENN, USA
Qian Wang	Shanghai Jiao Tong University, China
Rolf Heckemann	Sahlgrenska University Hospital, Sweden
Shaoting Zhang	UNC Charlotte, USA
Shu Liao	Siemens, USA
Simon Eskildsen	Center of Functionally Integrative Neuroscience, Denmark
Tobias Klinder	Philips, The Netherlands
Vladimir Fonov	McGill, Canada
Weidong Cai	The University of Sydney, Australia
Yefeng Zheng	Siemens, USA
Yong Fan	UPENN, USA
Yonggang Shi	University of Southern California, USA
Zhu Xiaofeng	UNC Chapel Hill, USA

Contents

Multi-atlas Segmentation

4D Multi-atlas Label Fusion Using Longitudinal Images

Yuankai Huo[1(✉)], Susan M. Resnick[2], and Bennett A. Landman[1]

[1] Electrical Engineering, Vanderbilt University, Nashville, TN, USA
yuankai.huo@vanderbilt.edu

[2] Laboratory of Behavioral Neuroscience, National Institute on Aging, Baltimore, MD, USA

Abstract. Longitudinal reproducibility is an essential concern in automated medical image segmentation, yet has proven to be an elusive objective as manual brain structure tracings have shown more than 10% variability. To improve reproducibility, longitudinal segmentation (4D) approaches have been investigated to reconcile temporal variations with traditional 3D approaches. In the past decade, multi-atlas label fusion has become a state-of-the-art segmentation technique for 3D image and many efforts have been made to adapt it to a 4D longitudinal fashion. However, the previous methods were either limited by using application specified energy function (e.g., surface fusion and multi model fusion) or only considered temporal smoothness on two consecutive time points (t and t + 1) under sparsity assumption. Therefore, a 4D multi-atlas label fusion theory for general label fusion purpose and simultaneously considering temporal consistency on all time points is appealing. Herein, we propose a novel longitudinal label fusion algorithm, called 4D joint label fusion (4DJLF), to incorporate the temporal consistency modeling via non-local patch-intensity covariance models. The advantages of 4DJLF include: (1) 4DJLF is under the general label fusion framework by simultaneously incorporating the spatial and temporal covariance on all longitudinal time points. (2) The proposed algorithm is a longitudinal generalization of a leading joint label fusion method (JLF) that has proven adaptable to a wide variety of applications. (3) The spatial temporal consistency of atlases is modeled in a probabilistic model inspired from both voting based and statistical fusion. The proposed approach improves the consistency of the longitudinal segmentation while retaining sensitivity compared with original JLF approach using the same set of atlases. The method is available online in open-source.

1 Introduction

An essential challenge in volumetric (3D) image segmentation on longitudinal medical images is to ensure the temporal consistency while retaining sensitivity. Many efforts have been made to incorporate the temporal dimension into volumetric segmentation (4D). One family of 4D methods is to control the longitudinal variations during pre/post-processing [1]. Another family is to incorporate the longitudinal variations within segmentation methods [2]. In the past decade, multi-atlas segmentation (MAS) has been regarded as de facto standard segmentation method in 3D scenarios

© Springer International Publishing AG 2017
G. Wu et al. (Eds.): Patch-MI 2017, LNCS 10530, pp. 3–11, 2017.
DOI: 10.1007/978-3-319-67434-6_1

[3–5]. To improve the performance of 4D MAS for longitudinal data, several previous avenues have been explored [6–8]. However, these methods are restricted on surface labeling application, availability of multi-modal data, or only considering two consecutive time points (t and t + 1) while assuming the l1-norm sparsity of fusion weights. When more than two longitudinal target images are available, the more comprehensive strategy is to consider the spatial smoothness on all time points (Fig. 1).

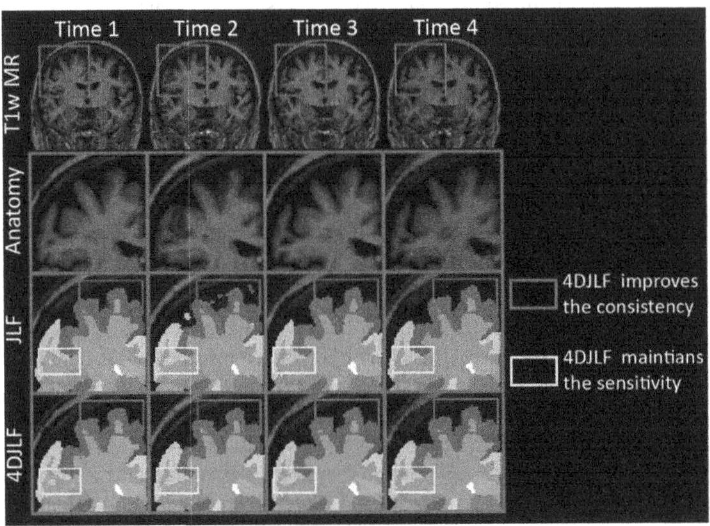

Fig. 1. An example of the inconsistency of 3D joint label fusion (JLF) segmentation across longitudinal multiple scans from the same subject. 4DJLF is proposed to improve the consistency while maintain the sensitivity.

In this paper, we propose a novel longitudinal label fusion algorithm, called 4D joint label fusion (4DJLF) to incorporate the probabilistic model of temporal performance of atlases to the voting based fusion. Briefly, we model the temporal performance of atlases on all time points in a probabilistic model and incorporate the leading and widely validated joint label fusion (JLF) framework.

2 Theory

2.1 Model Definition

A target image be represented by $T_t, t \in [1, 2, \ldots, k]$. 4DJLF considers all available longitudinal target images, $\mathbf{T} = \{T_1, T_2, \ldots, T_k\}$ where T_t represents a target image. First, all longitudinal target images are registered to the first-time point using rigid registration [9]. n pairs of atlases (one intensity atlas and one label atlas) $\mathbf{A} = \{A_1, A_2, \ldots, A_n\}$ are used in the MAS. Then, we register the n intensity atlases to k longitudinal target images to achieve $m = n \times k$ registered pairs of atlases. For mathematical convenience, we concatenate all registered atlases (based on the sequence in $\mathbf{T}$) to derive m registered intensity atlases set $\mathbf{I}$ and m registered label atlases set $\mathbf{S}$ as

$$\begin{aligned}\mathbf{I} &= \{I_1^{(1)}, \ldots, I_n^{(1)}, I_{n+1}^{(2)}, \ldots, I_{2n}^{(2)}, \cdots, I_{2n+1}^{(k)}, \ldots, I_m^{(k)}\} \\ \mathbf{S} &= \{S_1^{(1)}, \ldots, S_n^{(1)}, S_{n+1}^{(2)}, \ldots, S_{2n}^{(2)}, \cdots, S_{2n+1}^{(k)}, \ldots, S_m^{(k)}\}\end{aligned} \tag{1}$$

where the superscripts "(•)"indicate to which target image that atlas was registered.

The k longitudinal target images provide m registered atlases, where each atlas corresponds to one time point (target image). The consensus segmentation $\bar{S}$ for voxel x on t_{th} target image is $\bar{S}^t(x) = \sum_{i=1}^m w_i^t(x)S_i(x) = \mathbf{w}^t(x) \cdot \mathbf{S}(x)$,where $\mathbf{w}^t(x) = \{w_1^t(x), w_2^t(x), \ldots, w_m^t(x)\}$ are spatially varying weights restricted by $\sum_{i=1}^m w_i^k(x) = 1$. Adopting [10], the error $\delta_i^t(x)$ made by atlas S_i on t_{th} target image in the binary segmentation is $\delta_i^t(x) = S_T^t(x) - S_i(x)$, where $S_T^t(x)$ is the hidden true segmentation. $\delta_i^t(x) = 0$ indicates the right decision is made, while $\delta_i^t(x) = -1$ or 1 means the wrong decision is made. Then, our purpose is to find a set of voting weights $\mathbf{w}^t(x)$ for each target image T_t that minimize the total expected error between the automated labeled image $\bar{S}^k$ and hidden true S_T^t, given by the following energy function

$$\begin{aligned} & E_{\delta_1^t(x),\ldots,\delta_m^t(x)}\left[\left(S_T^t(x) - \bar{S}^t(x)\right)^2 | \mathbf{T}, \mathbf{I}\right] \\ &= \sum_{i=1}^m \sum_{j=1}^m w_i^t(x) w_j^t(x) E_{\delta_i^t(x)\delta_j^t(x)}\left[\delta_i^t(x)\delta_j^t(x) | T_1, \ldots, T_k, I_1, \ldots, I_m\right] = \mathbf{w}_x^{t^T} \boldsymbol{M}_x^t \mathbf{w}_x^t \end{aligned} \tag{2}$$

where $\mathbf{w}_x^{t^T}$ is the transpose of vector $\mathbf{w}_x^t$ at voxel x. $\boldsymbol{M}_x^t$ is a $m \times m$ pairwise dependency matrix that $\boldsymbol{M}_x^t(i,j) = p(\delta_i^t(x)\delta_j^t(x) = 1 | T_1, \ldots, T_k, I_1, \ldots, I_m)$. Finally, the estimated weights $\hat{\mathbf{w}}_x^t$, which is our target, is derived by $\hat{\mathbf{w}}_x^t = \arg\min_{\mathbf{w}_x^t} \mathbf{w}_x^{t^T}(\boldsymbol{M}_x^t + \alpha \boldsymbol{I})\mathbf{w}_x^t$.

2.2 JLF-Multi

As a baseline, we consider to use simple temporal model (JLF-Multi) to perform the 4D label fusion. We assume that each target image in $\mathbf{T}$ contributes equally to the label fusion for target T_t. In this case, $\boldsymbol{M}_x^t(i,j)$ is can be approximated as

$$\boldsymbol{M}_x^t(i,j) \propto \sum_{y \in B(x)} \cdot |T_t(y) - I_i(\mathcal{N}_i(y))| \cdot |T_t(y) - I_j(\mathcal{N}_j(y))| \tag{3}$$

where the Σ improves the spatial smoothness by adding multiple voxels y in a patch neighborhood $B(x)$ (e.g., $2 \times 2 \times 2$ by default), and the non-local patch searching is conducted within a search neighborhood $\mathcal{N}(y)$ (e.g., $3 \times 3 \times 3$ by default).

2.3 4DJLF

In JLF-Multi, each longitudinal target image contributes equally to the 4D label fusion. However, this assumption is not always valid. Herein, we propose the new dependency matrix $\ddot{\boldsymbol{M}}_x^t(i,j)$ by adaptively evaluating the longitudinal raters' performance on any target image patches using a probabilistic model

$$\ddot{\boldsymbol{M}}_{\boldsymbol{x}}^{\boldsymbol{t}}(i,j) = p\big(T_q(x), T_r(x)|T_t(x)\big) \cdot \Big(\sum\nolimits_{y\in B(x)} \Big|T_q(y) - I_i^{(q)}(\mathcal{N}_i(y))\Big| \cdot \Big|T_r(y) - I_j^{(r)}(\mathcal{N}_j(y))\Big|\Big) \tag{4}$$

where the new dependency matrix $\ddot{\boldsymbol{M}}_{\boldsymbol{x}}^{\boldsymbol{t}}(i,j)$ not only evaluates the similarity between atlases and target images but also considers the longitudinal similarities between target images. The "(q)" and "(r)" indicate which atlases that I_i and I_j were registered to and the value of q and r are derived from Eq. (1). Then, probability of using the raters (atlases) from T_{q} and T_{r} given target T_t is modeled in a conditional probability

$$p\big(T_q(x), T_r(x)|T_t(x)\big) = p\big(T_q(x)|T_t(x)\big) \cdot p\big(T_r(x)|T_t(x)\big) \tag{5}$$

by assuming T_{q} and T_{r} are conditionally independent, we have

$$p\big(\big(T_q(x)|T_t(x)\big)\big) = \exp\left(\beta \cdot \sum\nolimits_{y\in B(x)} \frac{|T_q(y) - T_t(y)|}{\Big|T_q(y) - I_i^{(q)}(\mathcal{N}_i(y))\Big|}\right) \tag{6}$$

$$p((T_r(x)|T_t(x))) = \exp\left(\beta \cdot \sum\nolimits_{y\in B(x)} \frac{|T_r(y) - T_t(y)|}{\Big|T_r(y) - I_j^{(r)}(\mathcal{N}_j(y))\Big|}\right) \tag{7}$$

where β is a sensitivity coefficient and is empirically set to 100 in the experiments.

2.4 Relationship Between 4DJLF to JLF

The proposed 4DJLF theory is a generalization of JLF. If the β is set to a large number, the $p\big(T_q(x), T_r(x)|T_t(x)\big)$ will be large for atlases from other time points, but still equals to 1 for the atlases from the target image itself. Therefore, the weights of the atlases from other time points will be close to zero and essentially only the atlases registered to the target time T_t are considered. In that case, 4DJLF degenerates to JLF. To see the relationship in Fig. 2, we redefine the right side of Eq. (5).

$$\Gamma_x(i,j) = \sum\nolimits_{y\in B(x)} \cdot \Big|T_q(y) - I_i^{(q)}(\mathcal{N}_i(y))\Big| \cdot \Big|T_r(y) - I_j^{(r)}(\mathcal{N}_j(y))\Big| \tag{8}$$

Then, we define a matrix $\Phi_{p,q}$ as the following

$$\Phi_x(q,r) = \begin{bmatrix} \Gamma_x(i',j') & \Gamma_x(i',j'+1) & \cdots & \Gamma_x(i',j'+k) \\ \Gamma_x(i'+1,j') & \Gamma_x(i'+1,j'+1) & & \Gamma_x(i'+1,j'+k) \\ & \vdots & \ddots & \vdots \\ \Gamma_x(i'+k,j') & \Gamma_x(i'+k,j'+1) & \cdots & \Gamma_x(i'+k,j'+k) \end{bmatrix} \tag{9}$$

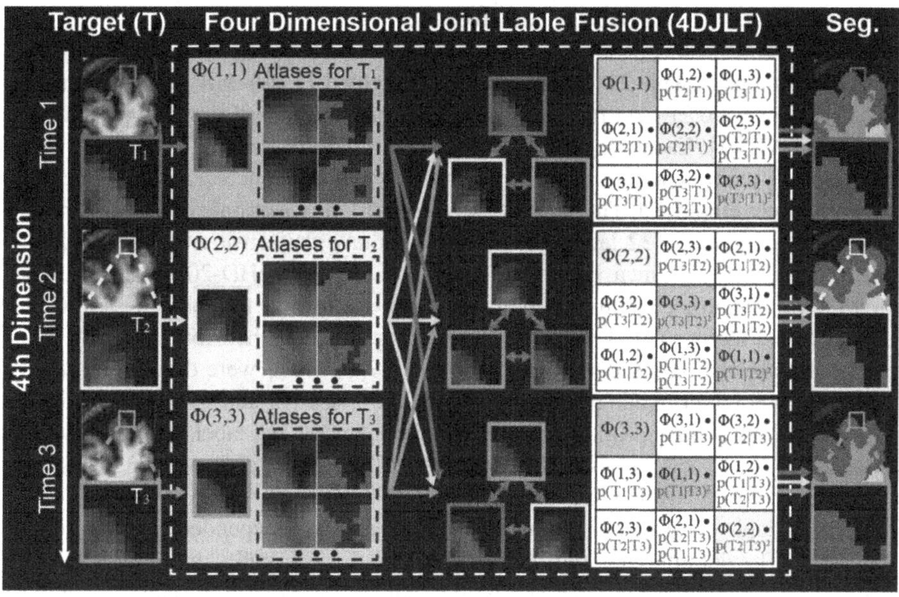

Fig. 2. The 4DJLF framework. First, the same set of atlases are registered to the longitudinal target images (3 time points in figure). Then, the Φ matrices are calculated using Eq. (9). Finally, the spatial temporal performance of all atlases are model by Eq. (10), which leads to the final segmentations ("Seg."). Note that the upper right 3×3 matrix is identical to Eq. (11). The original JLF estimates the block diagonal elements of the generalized covariance matrix (highlighted in magenta, green, and yellow) which would result in independent temporal estimates. (Color figure online)

where $i' = (q-1) \times k + 1$ and $j' = (r-1) \times k + 1$. For simplify, we assume three longitudinal target images are used and the first time point is the target image (upper row in Fig. 2). We rewrite the $p\left(\left(T_q(x)|T_t(x)\right)\right)$ as $p_x\left(\frac{T_q}{T_t}\right)$ to visualize the $\ddot{\boldsymbol{M}}^t$ at the first time point ($t = 1$ and the subscript x is omitted for simplicity). Since $p\left(\frac{T_1}{T_1}\right) = 1$, the $\ddot{\boldsymbol{M}}^1$ is further simplified to

$$\ddot{\boldsymbol{M}}^1 = \begin{bmatrix} \Phi(1,1) & \Phi(1,2)p\left(\frac{T_2}{T_1}\right) & \Phi(1,3)p\left(\frac{T_3}{T_1}\right) \\ \Phi(2,1)p\left(\frac{T_2}{T_1}\right) & \Phi(2,2)p\left(\frac{T_2}{T_1}\right)^2 & \Phi(2,3)p\left(\frac{T_2}{T_1}\right)p\left(\frac{T_3}{T_1}\right) \\ \Phi(3,1)p\left(\frac{T_3}{T_1}\right) & \Phi(3,2)p\left(\frac{T_3}{T_1}\right)p\left(\frac{T_2}{T_1}\right) & \Phi(3,3)p\left(\frac{T_3}{T_1}\right)^2 \end{bmatrix} \tag{10}$$

where $\ddot{\boldsymbol{M}}^1$ is identical to the upper right matrix in Fig. 2. Note that $\Phi(1,1)$ is the same as the M_x in JLF [10], which demonstrates the relationship between 4DJLF and JLF.

3 Experimental Methods and Results

Six healthy subjects with 21 longitudinal T1-weighted (T1w) MR scans (mean age 82.3, range: 72.5–90.2) were randomly selected from Baltimore Longitudinal Study of Aging (BLSA) [11]. Each image had 170 × 256 × 256 voxels with 1.2 × 1 × 1 mm resolution. 15 pairs of atlases from BrainCOLOR (http://braincolor.mindboggle.info/protocols/) were employed. The intensity atlases had 1 mm isotropic resolution and the label atlases contained 132 labels. In order to evaluate the sensitivity, one randomly selected T1w image from a healthy subject (age 11) in ADHD-200 OHSU dataset (http://fcon_1000.projects.nitrc.org/indi/adhd200/) was used in the robustness test. The 21 longitudinal target images were first affinely registered to the MNI305 atlas. Then, the spatially aligned longitudinal atlases $\mathbf{T} = \{T_1, T_2, \ldots, T_k\}$ were derived by rigidly registering each target image to the first time point. Then, 15 atlases were non-rigidly registered [12] to all target images to achieve the intensity and label atlases in Eq. (1) (performed $m = 15 \times 21$ non-rigid registrations). The same preprocessing was also deployed to the one ADHD-200 target image.

JLF was deployed on all 21 longitudinal target images independently using default parameters. The longitudinal reproducibility of JLF, JLF-multi and 4D JLF were evaluated by calculating the Dice similarity coefficients between all pairs of longitudinal images (Fig. 3a) Wilcoxon signed rank test and Cohen's d effect size were performed on JLF-Multi vs. JLF and 4D JLF vs. JLF. The "*" indicated the difference satisfied (1) $p < 0.01$ in Wilcoxon signed rank test, and (2) $d > 0.1$ in effect size. The temporal changes on volume sizes of whole brain, gray matter and white matter were shown in Fig. 4. Figure 5 shown the qualitative results from subject 5 in Fig. 4.

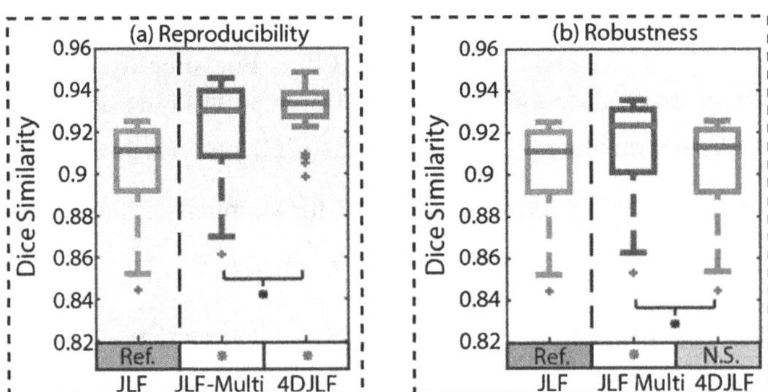

Fig. 3. Quantitative results. (a) The reproducibility experiment shown that the proposed 4DJLF had overall significantly better reproducibility than JLF and JLF-Multi. (b) The robustness test indicated that 4DJLF maintained the sensitivity as JLF, while JLF-Multi was not able to do so. The red "*" means the method satisfied both $p < 0.01$ and effect size > 0.1 compared with JLF ("Ref."), while the "N.S." means at least one was not satisfied. The black "*" means the difference between two methods satisfied both $p < 0.01$ and effect size > 0.1. (Color figure online)

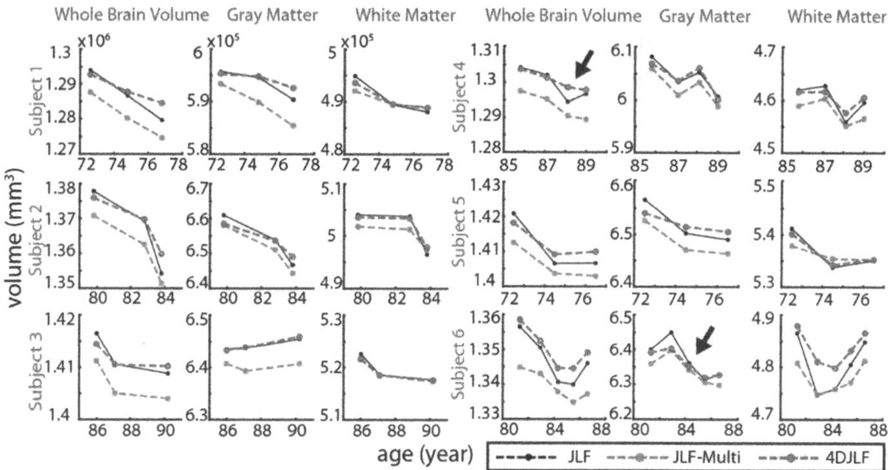

Fig. 4. This figure presents the longitudinal changes of whole brain volume, gray matter volume and white matter volume for all 6 subjects (21 time points). The black arrows indicate that the proposed 4DJLF reconciles some obvious temporal inconsistency by simultaneously considering all available longitudinal images.

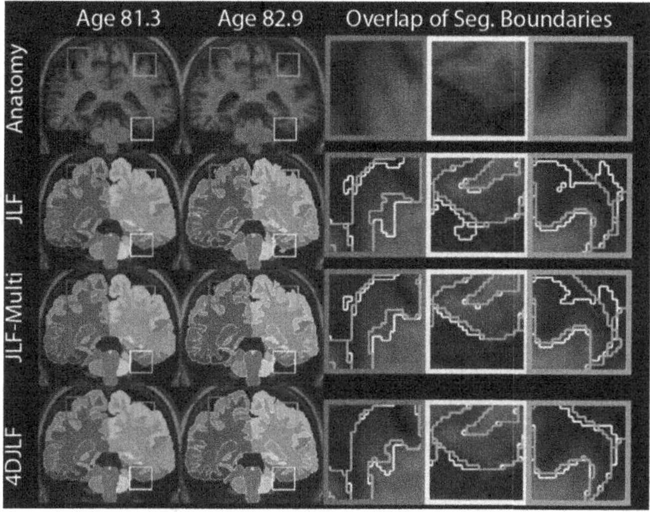

Fig. 5. Qualitative results of deploying longitudinal segmentation methods on two examples.

Second, a robustness test was conducted to evaluate the sensitivity of JLF, JLF-Multi and 4DJLF. We combined the previously mentioned ADHD-200 image to each target image to formed 21 dummy longitudinal pairs. This test simulated the large temporal variations since the two images in each pair were independent and collected from different scanners. Then, the 4D segmentation methods were deployed on such cases to see if the 4D methods can maintain the sensitivity compared with JLF. The Fig. 3b indicated the 4DJLF had "trivial" changes on reproducibility (effect size < 0.1) compared with JLF, while JLF-Multi had large differences compared with JLF.

4 Conclusion

We propose the 4DJLF multi-atlas label fusion strategy by modeling the spatial temporal performance of atlases. The proposed theory incorporates the ideas from the two major families of label fusion theories (voting based fusion and statistical fusion) by generalizing the JLF label fusion method to a 4D manner. The results demonstrated that the proposed method was not only able to improve the longitudinal reproducibility (Figs. 3a, 4 and 5) but also reduces the segmentation errors compared with traditional 3D JLF (Fig. 5). Meanwhile, the 4DJLF did not significantly change the segmentation reproducibility when performing on dummy longitudinal pairs of images (Fig. 3b).

Acknowledgments. This research was supported by NSF CAREER 1452485, NIH 5R21EY024 036, NIH 1R21NS064534, NIH 2R01EB006136, NIH 1R03EB012461, and supported by the Intramural Research Program, National Institute on Aging, NIH. This project was supported in part by the National Center for Research Resources, Grant UL1 RR024975-01, and is now at the National Center for Advancing Translational Sciences, Grant 2 UL1 TR000445-06. The content is solely the responsibility of the authors and does not necessarily represent the official views of the NIH.

References

1. Roy, S., Carass, A., Pacheco, J., Bilgel, M., Resnick, S.M., Prince, J.L., Pham, D.L.: Temporal filtering of longitudinal brain magnetic resonance images for consistent segmentation. NeuroImage Clin. **11**, 264–275 (2016)
2. Pham, D.L.: Spatial models for fuzzy clustering. Comput. Vis. Image Underst. **84**, 285–297 (2001)
3. Iglesias, J.E., Sabuncu, M.R.: Multi-atlas segmentation of biomedical images: a survey. Med. Image Anal. **24**, 205–219 (2015)
4. Huo, Y., Asman, A.J., Plassard, A.J., Landman, B.A.: Simultaneous total intracranial volume and posterior fossa volume estimation using multi-atlas label fusion. Hum. Brain Mapp. **38**, 599–616 (2017)
5. Huo, Y., Plassard, A.J., Carass, A., Resnick, S.M., Pham, D.L., Prince, J.L., Landman, B.A.: Consistent cortical reconstruction and multi-atlas brain segmentation. NeuroImage **138**, 197–210 (2016)
6. Li, G., Wang, L., Shi, F., Lin, W., Shen, D.: Multi-atlas based simultaneous labeling of longitudinal dynamic cortical surfaces in infants. In: Mori, K., Sakuma, I., Sato, Y., Barillot, C., Navab, N. (eds.) MICCAI 2013. LNCS, vol. 8149, pp. 58–65. Springer, Heidelberg (2013). doi:10.1007/978-3-642-40811-3_8
7. Guo, Y., Wu, G., Yap, P.-T., Jewells, V., Lin, W., Shen, D.: Segmentation of infant hippocampus using common feature representations learned for multimodal longitudinal data. In: Navab, N., Hornegger, J., Wells, William M., Frangi, Alejandro F. (eds.) MICCAI 2015. LNCS, vol. 9351, pp. 63–71. Springer, Cham (2015). doi:10.1007/978-3-319-24574-4_8

8. Wang, L., Guo, Y., Cao, X., Wu, G., Shen, D.: Consistent multi-atlas hippocampus segmentation for longitudinal MR brain images with temporal sparse representation. In: Wu, G., Coupé, P., Zhan, Y., Munsell, Brent C., Rueckert, D. (eds.) Patch-MI 2016. LNCS, vol. 9993, pp. 34–42. Springer, Cham (2016). doi:10.1007/978-3-319-47118-1_5
9. Ourselin, S., Roche, A., Subsol, G., Pennec, X., Ayache, N.: Reconstructing a 3D structure from serial histological sections. Image Vis. Comput. **19**, 25–31 (2001)
10. Wang, H.Z., Suh, J.W., Das, S.R., Pluta, J.B., Craige, C., Yushkevich, P.A.: Multi-atlas segmentation with joint label fusion. IEEE Trans. Pattern Anal. **35**, 611–623 (2013)
11. Resnick, S.M., Pham, D.L., Kraut, M.A., Zonderman, A.B., Davatzikos, C.: Longitudinal magnetic resonance imaging studies of older adults: a shrinking brain. J. Neurosci.: Off. J. Soc. Neurosci. **23**, 3295–3301 (2003)
12. Avants, B.B., Epstein, C.L., Grossman, M., Gee, J.C.: Symmetric diffeomorphic image registration with cross-correlation: evaluating automated labeling of elderly and neurodegenerative brain. Med. Image Anal. **12**, 26–41 (2008)

Brain Image Labeling Using Multi-atlas Guided 3D Fully Convolutional Networks

Longwei Fang[1,2,4], Lichi Zhang[4], Dong Nie[4], Xiaohuan Cao[4,5], Khosro Bahrami[4], Huiguang He[1,2,3(✉)], and Dinggang Shen[4(✉)]

[1] Research Center for Brain-Inspired Intelligence, Institute of Automation, Chinese Academy of Sciences, Beijing, China
huiguang.he@ia.ac.cn
[2] University of Chinese Academy of Sciences, Beijing, China
[3] Center for Excellence in Brain Science and Intelligence Technology, Chinese Academy of Sciences, Beijing, China
[4] Department of Radiology and BRIC, University of North Carolina at Chapel Hill, Chapel Hill, NC, USA
dinggang_shen@med.unc.edu
[5] School of Automation, Northwestern Polytechnical University, Xi'an, China

Abstract. Automatic labeling of anatomical structures in brain images plays an important role in neuroimaging analysis. Among all methods, multi-atlas based segmentation methods are widely used, due to their robustness in propagating prior label information. However, non-linear registration is always needed, which is time-consuming. Alternatively, the patch-based methods have been proposed to relax the requirement of image registration, but the labeling is often determined independently by the target image information, without getting direct assistance from the atlases. To address these limitations, in this paper, we propose a multi-atlas guided 3D fully convolutional networks (FCN) for brain image labeling. Specifically, multi-atlas based guidance is incorporated during the network learning. Based on this, the discriminative of the FCN is boosted, which eventually contribute to accurate prediction. Experiments show that the use of multi-atlas guidance improves the brain labeling performance.

1 Introduction

Accurate labeling of neuro-anatomical regions is highly demanded for quantitative analysis of MR brain images. Many attempts have been made in automatic labeling methods since it is infeasible to manually label a large set of 3D MR images. However, it remains a challenging problem due to the complicated brain structures and also the ambiguous boundaries between some regions of interest (ROIs).

The multi-atlas based methods have emerged as the standard way in the brain image labeling for its effectiveness and robustness. By using the atlases, each with a single MRI scan and its manual label maps, the multi-atlas based methods first *register* multiple atlases to the target image and then *fuse* the respective deformed atlas label maps to obtain the labeling results. Many relevant works have been made to improve the performances of these *registration* and *label fusion* steps in the multi-atlas based

© Springer International Publishing AG 2017
G. Wu et al. (Eds.): Patch-MI 2017, LNCS 10530, pp. 12–19, 2017.
DOI: 10.1007/978-3-319-67434-6_2

methods, as summarized in [1–3]. However, one major limitation of these multi-atlas based method is that it always needs non-rigid registration for aligning atlases to the subject, which is time-consuming [4]. Besides, it is also a challenging work to obtain accurate registration, which will eventually affect the final labeling performance.

On the other hand, the patch-based methods have gained increased attentions recently, which are mainly developed to relax the high demands of registration accuracy in the multi-atlas based methods. Specifically, in the patch-based methods, each patch in the target subject image looks for its similar patches in the atlas images according to patch similarity. Then, the label of those selected atlas patches are fused together to label the center voxel of subject patch [5, 6]. The weights of selected atlas patches in the label fusion process are estimated based on their intensity similarity with the target subject patch. Also, Wu et al. [7] further proposed using a multi-scale feature representation and label-specific patch partition method to extend the label fusion strategy. In this method, each patch is represented by the multi-scale features that encode both local and semi-local image information, and then the image patch is further partitioned into a set of label specific partial image patches. Finally, the hierarchical patch-based label fusion is followed to finish the labeling. On the other hand, the learning-based methods have also been incorporated into the brain image labeling process, generally in a patch-based manner. For example, Tu and Bai [8] extracted the 3D Haar features from the atlases and then employed the probabilistic boosting tree (PBT) to learn the classifier for brain labeling. Hao et al. [9] introduced a hippocampus segmentation method using L1-regularized support vector machine (SVM), with a k-nearest neighbor (kNN) based training sample strategy. Moreover, the random forest has also been widely applied, since it can efficiently handle a large number of training atlases, and can largely avoid the overfitting problem in the conventional decision tree methods by incorporating the uniform bagging strategy [10, 11]. Recently, fully convolutional networks (FCN) [12] have shown excellent performance in natural image segmentation and recognition. Some researchers have also employed the FCN model for medical image segmentation. For example, Nie et al. [13] adopted the FCN model for brain tissue segmentation, which has shown a promising result.

However, the main limitation of the current methods is that they determine the target labels merely on the local appearance of target image patch, without considering the direct label information from those similar atlas patches. Besides, although patch-based methods can relax the demand of accurate registration, most methods [6–10] still apply *non-rigid* registration to preprocessing the data, for the benefit of labeling improvements.

In this paper, we intend to solve the aforementioned issues by proposing a multi-atlas guided 3D FCN model for improving the performance of brain labeling. The major contribution here is two-fold. *First*, we develop a novel multi-atlas guidance strategy, which can directly utilize prior information in the atlases to guide and improve the labeling capability. *Second*, different from the conventional multi-atlas based methods, we need no *non-rigid* registration for aligning atlases to the target image, by still guaranteeing the reasonable labeling performance. This will greatly reduce the time cost for the overall labeling process, thus making it more applicable for future clinical applications.

2 Methods

In this section, we will illustrate the details of our proposed multi-atlas guided FCN method, which consists of the *training* and *testing* stages. In the *training* stage, we first select a number of images from the training set, and consider them as the atlas images. Then, we extract 3D cubic patches from the training images, and, for each selected training patch, we also select K most similar atlas patches from the linearly-aligned atlas images. Next, each training patch and its corresponding selected atlas patches (including intensity patches and label patches) are used together to train the FCN model. In the *testing* stage, the trained FCN model is first applied to each input testing patch (of the new testing image) and its selected atlas patches, for obtaining a predicted label patch. Then, all the predicted label patches from all locations of the testing image are fused together to give the final labeling result.

2.1 Training Data Preparation

Data Preprocessing: The first step is normalizing the intensity of data in the range from 0 to 255. And before the patch extraction process, for each training image, we first register all atlases to its space. As stated above, we need no *non-rigid* registration; instead, we just use affine registration, which can be implemented more efficiently. Specifically, we first linearly align the intensity images of atlases to the target training image using the *flirt* in FSL [14], and warp the label maps of all atlases to the training image space by using the obtained respective linear transformation for each atlas.

Patch Extraction: Since there are high variations of ROI sizes for different brain ROIs under labeling, we develop a specific patch extraction strategy to ensure that the sufficient training patches can be extracted from each ROI under labeling. Specifically, this strategy ensures an adequate number of patches extracted around the boundary of each ROI, since boundaries contain the direct shape information vital for ROI labeling. To do this, we first employ a canny edge detector to find boundaries in each of the atlas label maps. Then, we randomly select the patches by ensuring that (1) the number of patches extracted from every ROI is similar, and (2) the number of patches extracted from the boundary of each ROI is similar to the number of patches extracted from internal part of each ROI.

Atlas Patch Selection: For each given training image patch $P_{T(I,j)}$, centered at voxel j and extracted from the training image I, we can find one most similar atlas image patch from each atlas in the 3D cubic searching neighborhood $c(j)$, i.e., according to the image intensity similarity. This step can be mathematically summarized by Eq. 1, where (M, n) is an atlas image patch selected from the atlas image at the location of voxel n, and $||\cdot||_2$ is a Euclidean distance measure between image patches under comparison.

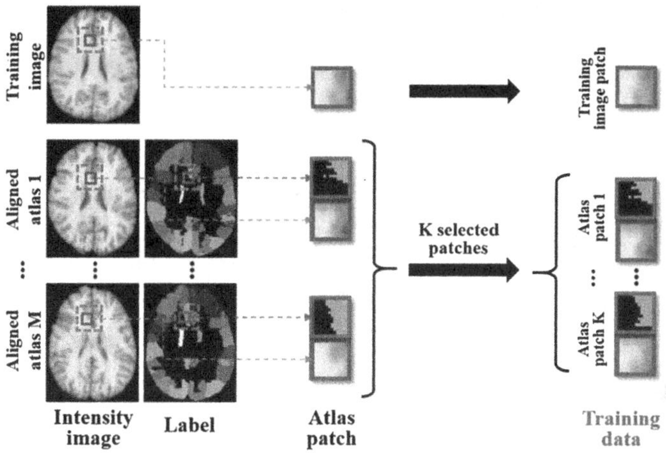

Fig. 1. A brief illustration of steps for preparing the training data. The green dash box is the searching neighborhood. (Color figure online)

$$\hat{P} = \{P_{A(M,n)} | \min_{n \in c(j)} ||P_{T(I,j)} - P_{A(M,n)}||_2^2\} \tag{1}$$

By ranking all the selected atlas image patches according to their respective similarities to the training image patch $(I,)$, we can finally select the top K (i.e., $K = 3$) atlas image patches. Then, each training image patch and its K selected atlas image patches are combined as joint input to train our proposed FCN model. Figure 1 summaries all steps in our method for prepressing the training data to train the FCN model.

2.2 Fully Convolutional Networks (FCN) Configuration

We employ an FCN model for the brain ROI labeling. FCN model is an end-to-end learning structure, with its output as a patch. Compared with the convolutional neural networks (CNN) [16] that output is just the label for the center voxel of the input image patch, FCN can label the whole patch in one process, thus more efficient and potentially more spatially-consistent labeling than CNN. The configuration of our FCN (as shown in Fig. 2) is briefed below. (1) We first learn $K + 1$ mapping structures separately for the training image patch and K selected atlas image/label patches. Specifically, in the first layer, for each of K sets of selected atlas image/label patches, we use K concatenated layers to group the image patch and label patch of the same atlas together. For the training image patch, since there is no label patch, it is simply input the FCN. Next, three convolution layers are applied to each of $K + 1$ mapping structures, followed by a max pooling layer for down sampling the mapped data. (2) After separately mapping the training image patch and the K selected atlas image/label patches, we use another concatenation layer to combine $K + 1$ sets of mapped data together, followed by two

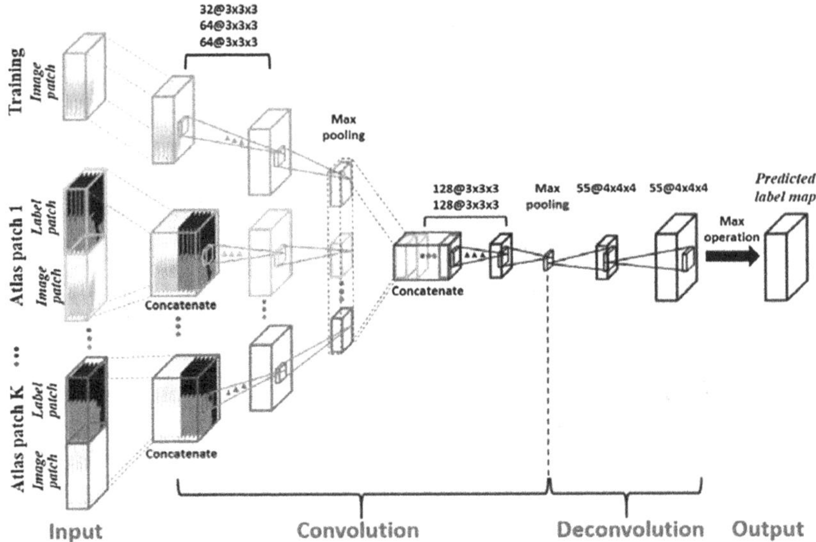

Fig. 2. Detailed structure and parameters of our proposed FCN model for patch labeling.

convolution layers and a max pooling layer. (3) Finally, we use two deconvolution layers to get the label map. Note that the rectified linear units (ReLU) is used as our activation function for all the convolution layers, and also cross-entropy loss is used as our loss function.

2.3 Brain Labeling

For each new testing brain image, we first use affine registration to align all the atlases to this target image. Then, for each (testing) image patch (with the same size as all the training image patches) extracted from the testing image, we select its *K* most similar atlas image patches from all linearly-aligned atlases as described in Sect. 2.1. Next, each testing image patch and its *K* selected atlas image/label patches are combined and inputted to our trained FCN for obtained the patch labeling result. Finally, the labeling results from all testing patches covering the whole testing image are fused together (with majority voting) to produce a final label map for the testing image.

3 Experimental Results

We use the LONI LPBA40[1] dataset to evaluate the performance of our proposed brain ROI labeling method. The LONI LPBA40 dataset contains 40 T1-weighted MR brain images with 54 manually labeled ROIs. In our method, four-fold cross validation is

[1] http://www.loni.ucla.edu/Atlases/LPBA40.

used. Specifically, in each fold, we select 10 images as the testing images, and the rest as the training images. Furthermore, we select 10 images from those 30 training images as the atlas images, and other 2 images as the validation images for FCN training. Note that we also train another FCN model without using multi-atlas guidance (i.e., just using the training image patch), and use it as the baseline method. Note that the network structures and parameters are same in both our proposed multi-atlas guided FCN method and this baseline method. In our paper, we use the patch size of $24 \times 24 \times 24$ in voxels, and the searching neighborhood size of $30 \times 30 \times 30$ also in voxels. The number of training image patches sampled from each training image is 8,400. For the testing image, we evenly visit patches with a step size of 9 voxels, to ensure a sufficient overlap for the neighboring patches.

We evaluate the labeling performance using the Dice Similarity Coefficient (DSC). The results on LONI LPBA40 show that our proposed method can achieve the average DSC of $(80.33 \pm 1.26)\%$ for 54 ROIs. Table 1 lists the comparison of our method with the state-of-art methods. Note that, for these state-of-art methods, we simply copied results from [7, 10, 11] for fair comparison. It can be observed that our proposed method outperforms the non-local based method [11] for more than 2%, and also achieves a comparable labeling results to the non-rigid registration methods [7, 10]. Although the mean DSC estimations by the multi-atlas method [10] and our proposed method are close, it can be observed that our method has a much smaller standard deviation, suggesting that our method is more reliable. Furthermore, it often takes 2–20 h for just the non-rigid registration step in multi-atlas method [15], while our proposed method takes less than 15 min for labeling a testing image which is definitely more efficient in the application stage.

Table 1. Quantitative comparison between the proposed method and the state-of-arts methods.

Method	Non-rigid registration		Affine registration		
	Multi-atlases [7]	Learning [10]	Non-local [11]	FCN-single patch	Proposed
DSC (%)	81.46 ± 2.25	80.1 ± 4.53	78.26 ± 4.83	78.20 ± 1.60	80.33 ± 1.26

We further compared our method with the baseline method (namely FCN-single patch) in Table 1, which shows significant improvements for ROI labeling using multi-atlas guidance in our method. The structure of baseline method is similar with proposed method, except that baseline method does not have atlas patches. Figure 3 also shows a labeled testing image by the baseline method (FCN-single patch) and our proposed method (Proposed). Figure 3(a) shows the golden standard (obtained with manual delineation). Figure 3(b) shows the labeling result by the baseline method (FCN-single patch), and Fig. 3(c) shows the labeling result by our proposed method (Proposed). It can be observed that, the labeling results on the boundary by proposed method is smoother than the baseline method. Moreover, there are wrong predictions inside of some ROIs by the baseline method, as indicated in Fig. 3(b). When using multi-atlas guidance to train the FCN model in our proposed method, more prior labeling information from multiple atlases can be used to directly help refine the labeling results, thus avoiding the wrong labeling by the baseline method.

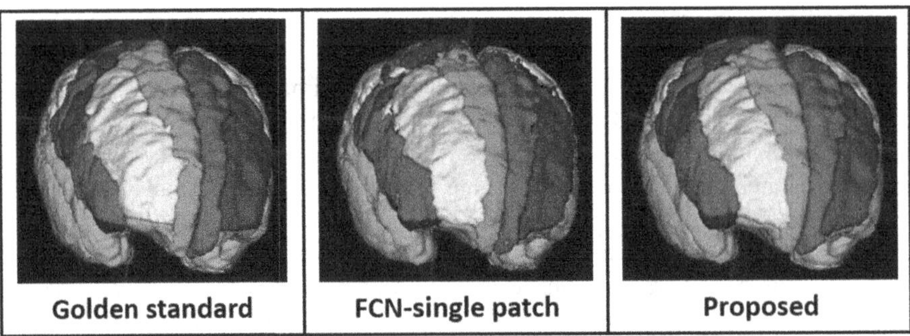

Fig. 3. Visual comparison of labeling results by the baseline method (FCN-single patch) and our proposed method (Proposed).

4 Conclusion

In this paper, we have presented a multi-atlas guided 3D FCN method for brain ROI labeling. Different from the traditional neural networks, the input to our FCN includes *not only* the intensity image patch from training (or testing) image, *but also* both the intensity and label patches from the atlases. Such combination can provide a clearer guidance for FCN to better label the target brain images. Furthermore, our proposed method requires no non-rigid registration for data preprocessing. The validation results on a public dataset show that our proposed method outperforms the non-local based methods in accuracy and non-registration based methods in speed, as well as the baseline method in terms of labeling accuracy.

References

1. Jia, H., Yap, P.T., Shen, D.: Iterative multi-atlas-based multi-image segmentation with tree-based registration. NeuroImage **59**(1), 422–430 (2012)
2. Wolz, R., Aljabar, P., Hajnal, J.V., Hammers, A., Rueckert, D., The Alzheimer's Disease Neuroimaging Initiative: LEAP: learning embeddings for atlas propagation. NeuroImage **49** (2), 1316–1325 (2010)
3. Langerak, T.R., van der Heide, U.A., Kotte, A.N., Viergever, M.A., Van Vulpen, M., Pluim, J.P.: Label fusion in atlas-based segmentation using a selective and iterative method for performance level estimation (SIMPLE). IEEE Trans. Med. Imaging **29**(12), 2000–2008 (2010)
4. Iglesias, J.E., Sabuncu, M.R.: Multi-atlas segmentation of biomedical images: a survey. Med. Image Anal. **24**(1), 205–219 (2015)
5. Coupé, P., Manjón, J.V., Fonov, V., Pruessner, J., Robles, M., Collins, D.L.: Patchbased segmentation using expert priors: application to hippocampus and ventricle segmentation. NeuroImage **54**(2), 940–954 (2011)
6. Wang, H., Suh, J.W., Das, S.R., Pluta, J.B., Craige, C., Yushkevich, P.A.: Multiatlas segmentation with joint label fusion. IEEE Trans. Pattern Anal. Mach. Intell. **35**(3), 611–623 (2013)

7. Wu, G., Kim, M., Sanroma, G., Wang, Q., Munsell, B.C., Shen, D., The Alzheimer's Disease Neuroimaging Initiative: Hierarchical multi-atlas label fusion with multi-scale feature representation and labelspecific patch partition. NeuroImage **106**, 34–46 (2015)
8. Tu, Z., Bai, X.: Auto-context and its application to high-level vision tasks and 3D brain image segmentation. IEEE Trans. Pattern Anal. Mach. Intell. **32**(10), 1744–1757 (2010)
9. Hao, Y., Wang, T., Zhang, X., Duan, Y., Yu, C., Jiang, T., Fan, Y.: Local label learning (LLL) for subcortical structure segmentation: application to hippocampus segmentation. Hum. Brain Mapp. **35**(6), 2674–2697 (2014)
10. Zikic, D., Glocker, B., Criminisi, A.: Encoding atlases by randomized classification forests for efficient multi-atlas label propagation. Med. Image Anal. **18**(8), 1262–1273 (2014)
11. Zhang, L., Wang, Q., Gao, Y., Wu, G., Shen, D.: Automatic labeling of MR brain images by hierarchical learning of atlas forests. Med. Phys. **43**(3), 1175–1186 (2016)
12. Long, J., Shelhamer, E., Darrell, T.: Fully convolutional networks for semantic segmentation. In: Proceedings of the IEEE Conference on Computer Vision and Pattern Recognition, pp. 3431–3440 (2015)
13. Nie, D., Wang, L., Gao, Y., Sken, D.: Fully convolutional networks for multimodality isointense infant brain image segmentation. In: 2016 IEEE 13th International Symposium on Biomedical Imaging (ISBI), pp. 1342–1345. IEEE (2016)
14. Woolrich, M.W., Jbabdi, S., Patenaude, B., Chappell, M., Makni, S., Behrens, T., Beckmann, C., Jenkinson, M., Smith, S.M.: Bayesian analysis of neuroimaging data in FSL. Neuroimage **45**(1), S173–S186 (2009)
15. Landman, B., Warfield, S.: Miccai 2012 workshop on multi-atlas labeling. In: Medical Image Computing and Computer Assisted Intervention Conference 2012: MICCAI 2012 Grand Challenge and Workshop on Multi-Atlas Labeling Challenge Results (2012)
16. Moeskops, P., Viergever, M.A., Mendrik, A.M., de Vries, L.S., Benders, M.J., I˘sgum, I.: Automatic segmentation of MR brain images with a convolutional neural network. IEEE Trans. Med. Imaging **35**(5), 1252–1261 (2016)

Whole Brain Parcellation with Pathology: Validation on Ventriculomegaly Patients

Aaron Carass[1,2(✉)], Muhan Shao[1], Xiang Li[1], Blake E. Dewey[1], Ari M. Blitz[3], Snehashis Roy[4], Dzung L. Pham[4], Jerry L. Prince[1,2], and Lotta M. Ellingsen[1,5]

[1] Department of Electrical and Computer Engineering, The Johns Hopkins University, Baltimore, MD 21218, USA
aaron_carass@jhu.edu

[2] Department of Computer Science, The Johns Hopkins University, Baltimore, MD 21218, USA

[3] Department of Radiology and Radiological Science, The Johns Hopkins University, Baltimore, MD 21287, USA

[4] CNRM, The Henry M. Jackson Foundation for the Advancement of Military Medicine, Bethesda, MD 20892, USA

[5] Department of Electrical and Computer Engineering, University of Iceland, Reykjavik, Iceland

Abstract. Numerous brain disorders are associated with ventriculomegaly; normal pressure hydrocephalus (NPH) is one example. NPH presents with dementia-like symptoms and is often misdiagnosed as Alzheimer's due to its chronic nature and nonspecific presenting symptoms. However, unlike other forms of dementia NPH can be treated surgically with an over 80% success rate on appropriately selected patients. Accurate assessment of the ventricles, in particular its sub-compartments, is required to diagnose the condition. Existing segmentation algorithms fail to accurately identify the ventricles in patients with such extreme pathology. We present an improvement to a whole brain segmentation approach that accurately identifies the ventricles and parcellates them into four sub-compartments. Our work is a combination of patch-based tissue segmentation and multi-atlas registration-based labeling. We include a validation on NPH patients, demonstrating superior performance against state-of-the-art methods.

Keywords: Brain · MRI · Enlarged ventricles · Hydrocephalus

1 Introduction

The ventricular system of the human brain is made up of four cavities: the left and right lateral ventricles and the third and fourth ventricles. These cavities are connected via narrow channels, with the foramina of Monro connecting each of the lateral ventricles with the third ventricle and the cerebral aqueduct connecting the third and fourth ventricles. Each of these cavities contain choroid plexus, which is responsible for producing cerebrospinal fluid (CSF). In a healthy

© Springer International Publishing AG 2017
G. Wu et al. (Eds.): Patch-MI 2017, LNCS 10530, pp. 20–28, 2017.
DOI: 10.1007/978-3-319-67434-6_3

system, CSF is allowed to flow from the lateral ventricles into the third and then the fourth ventricle and subsequently into the central canal of the spinal cord and up into the subarachnoid space, before passing through the arachnoid villi into the venous sinuses.

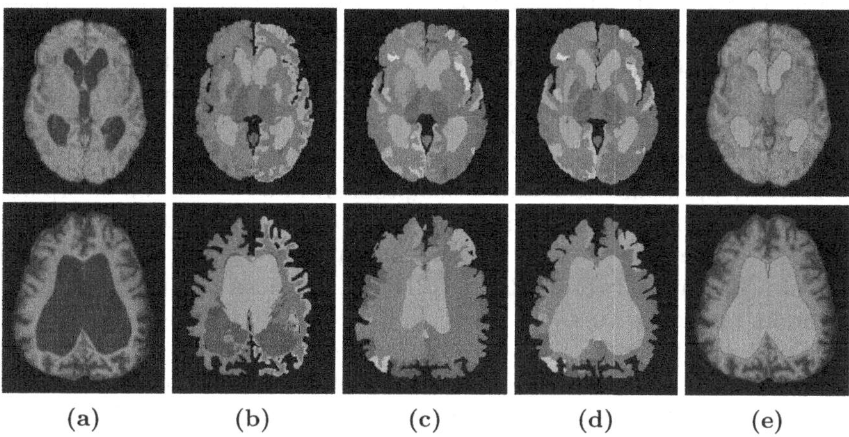

Fig. 1. Shown in each row is the (a) T_1-w MPRAGE of a NPH patient and the ventricle segmentation (green/cyan is the right/left lateral ventricle, blue is the 3rd ventricle) generated by (b) FreeSurfer [8], (c) MALPEM [9], (d) RUDOLPH, and (e) a manual delineation. The first row shows a NPH patient where all three algorithms performed well and the second row shows a more severe case where FreeSurfer and MALPEM have failed. The other colors show the rich tapestry of labels available in all three methods. (Color figure online)

Normal pressure hydrocephalus (NPH) is a disorder of the ventricular system caused by obstruction of the flow of CSF leading to the expansion of the cerebral ventricles and with symptoms including [1]: gait disturbance, urinary incontinence, and dementia. An example of a T_1-weighted (T_1-w) magnetization prepared rapid gradient echo (MPRAGE) of an NPH patient can be seen in Fig. 1(a). The expanded ventricular system presses against the surrounding structures causing the brain shape to become distorted and results in brain damage. NPH is routinely misdiagnosed as other forms of dementia, such as Parkinson's disease or Alzheimer's disease. However, unlike other forms of dementia, NPH is treatable and the associated symptoms can be reversed (to a certain extent) [10]. Treatment involves shunt surgery or endoscopic third ventriculostomy. However, diagnosing NPH patients is challenging using current methods, and the benefit of surgical intervention is sensitive to properly selected patients [14]. The chronically dilated ventricles are readily observed through magnetic resonance imaging (MRI), which when used in conjunction with a lumbar puncture and evaluation of the clinical response to removal of CSF can help to diagnose the condition. However, having accurate parcellation of the ventricular system into its sub-compartments would be of great clinical benefit to better characterize the pathology of NPH as well as to help in surgical planning, such that patients who will benefit from surgical treatments could be more robustly identified.

Previous work on ventricle segmentation [5,13] has focused on the ventricular system as one component of the brain. Newer methods [9] that provide an improved ventricle segmentation rely, in part, on multi-atlas segmentation frameworks, which enable them to identify some of the components of the ventricles (right and left lateral, 3rd, 4th) based on the labels available within their atlases. These more recent methods, however, often fail to correctly identify the extents of the ventricles in pathological cases, see Fig. 1. This occurs chiefly because they depend on a registration between the atlas and subject, which in pathological cases is rarely optimum. To address this problem in our work, we incorporate a patch-based segmentation method [11,12] to provide a prior for a multi-atlas label fusion framework [9]. Our method, known as robust dictionary-learning and label propagation hybrid (RUDOLPH) [7], provides a parcellation of the entire brain, providing 138 brain labels (in the cerebellum and cerebrum) while performing accurate ventricular segmentation even with enlarged ventricles. We present a detailed evaluation of this method with respect to the four main cavities of the ventricular system of NPH patients (noting that RUDOLPH also provides a parcellation of the whole brain, examples of which can be seen in Fig. 1). In Sect. 2, we describe RUDOLPH. Section 3 includes our experiments comparing our approach and two state-of-the-art segmentation algorithms on our manual delineations. We conclude with a discussion of the presented work in Sect. 4.

2 Method

The proposed method integrates the subject specific sparse dictionary learning (S3DL) method [11,12] and the multi-atlas label propagation with expectation-maximization (MALPEM) method [9]. S3DL is a patch-based segmentation method that uses sparse dictionary learning to classify the human brain into seven structures (cerebellar and cerebral white matter; cortical, subcortical, and cerebellar gray matter; and ventricular and cortical CSF). MALPEM is a multi-atlas label fusion scheme, which we modify to incorporate the seven labels from S3DL, intelligently guiding the multi-atlas label fusion framework. MALPEM cannot, in general, segment the ventricles in moderate to severe cases of NPH patients, due to the pathology (see Fig. 1(b)).

We first process a subject's MR image through S3DL. S3DL requires an atlas with its corresponding hard segmentation, and spatial priors depicting where the different tissues are expected to be located. The priors are computed using a simple blurring of the known atlas segmentation. S3DL adaptively modifies the subject priors to handle anatomical variability. The CSF labels from S3DL are incorporated within MALPEM, as described below.

We then register using SyN [2] 15 manually labeled atlases into the subject's space, with each atlas made up of 138 cortical and subcortical labels from

Neuromorphometrics[1]. This is similar to the first step of MALPEM, which uses 30 atlases. The output of this step is a probabilistic segmentation $\Pi = \{\pi_1, \ldots, \pi_n\}$, where π_i is a K-dimensional vector representing the $K = 138$ labels in the atlases, and n is the total number of voxels in the subject's image. MALPEM provides two label correction schemes; the first based on intensity-refined posterior probabilities, and the second relaxes the probabilities, Π, to correct for misregistration of the atlases. The eight CSF labels within Neuromorphometrics are assumed to come from the Gaussian distribution $(\mu_{\text{CSF}}, \sigma_{\text{CSF}})$ which is estimated based on Π. For each label k, $(k = 1, \ldots, K)$ we estimate (μ_k, σ_k) from the subject's image intensities. Then Π is relaxed to Π^R using the distributions (μ_k, σ_k) as follows. At each voxel i, a fraction α_{ik} of prior π_{ik} is redistributed from label k to one of the eight CSF labels based on the spatial proximity of the label to the CSF label with the highest probability. Both of these conditions fail in NPH patients since at the boundary of severely dilated ventricles the closest CSF label is usually cortical CSF and not the desired ventricular CSF and the severe deformation of NPH patients means that spatial information from anatomical atlases is incorrect.

To address this, we use the segmentation from S3DL. Thus, we identify the appropriate CSF label k_{CSF} as

$$k_{\text{CSF}} = \begin{cases} \underset{k \in \mathcal{C}_{\text{MALPEM}}}{\arg\max}\ \pi_{ik} & \text{if } \pi_{ik} \neq 0 \text{ for some } \\ & \quad k \in \mathcal{C}_{\text{MALPEM}}, \\ \underset{k \in \mathcal{C}_{\text{S3DL}}}{\arg\max}\ d_k(i) & \text{otherwise}, \end{cases} \tag{1}$$

where $d_k(i)$ is the distance from the voxel i to the nearest voxel with the current label k, and $\mathcal{C}_{\text{MALPEM}}$ and $\mathcal{C}_{\text{S3DL}}$ are the CSF labels of MALPEM and S3DL, respectively. We follow the MALPEM framework and compute the relaxation fraction, α_{ik}, based on the probability that the voxel x comes from either the intensity distribution $\mathcal{N}_k(x)$ estimated by label k or from one of the CSF distributions estimated by $\mathcal{N}_{k_{\text{CSF}}}(x)$,

$$\alpha_{ik} = \begin{cases} 0 & \mathcal{N}_k(x) \geq \mathcal{N}_{k_{\text{CSF}}}(x), \\ \max\left(0, \min\left(0.5 - \pi_{ik_{\text{CSF}}}, \pi_{ik}\right)\right) & \text{otherwise}. \end{cases} \tag{2}$$

The relaxed prior Π^R is computed as

$$\alpha_{ik}^R = \begin{cases} \pi_{ik} + \sum_{l \neq k_{\text{CSF}}} \alpha_{il} & \text{if } k = k_{\text{CSF}}, \\ \pi_{ik} - \alpha_{ik} & \text{otherwise}. \end{cases} \tag{3}$$

Π^R is then updated through an expectation-maximization framework [15], with smoothness of the final segmentation maintained through a Markov Random Field [17], which is the same as in the MALPEM framework.

[1] http://www.neuromorphometrics.com.

3 Results

Our data was acquired on a Siemens 3 T scanner using a T_1-w MPRAGE with TR = 10.3 ms, TE = 6 ms, and $0.82 \times 0.82 \times 1.17$ mm^3 voxel size. We processed a total of 45 NPH patients that were broadly classified based on the severity of their ventricular expansion into mild, moderate, and severe cases. All 45 NPH patients had their ventricular system manually delineated. This was done by identifying the anatomical structure of the ventricles, which required 3–4 h per patient. These were reviewed by separate experts in neuroanatomy, with possible correction or return to the delineator for correction. For 18 of the 45 NPH patients, once a ventricular system mask was agreed, the components of right and left lateral ventricles, both foramina of Monro, third ventricle, cerebral aqueduct, and fourth ventricle were identified. This parcellation of the ventricular system took another hour per patient to complete. The cerebral aqueduct and the foramina of Monro are not included within our validation as there do not currently exist such detailed anatomical atlases of the ventricular system in use elsewhere. Thus for validation purposes, the foramina of Monro is included with the corresponding lateral ventricle, and the cerebral aqueduct with the fourth ventricle, making the labeling comparable with Neuromorphometrics.

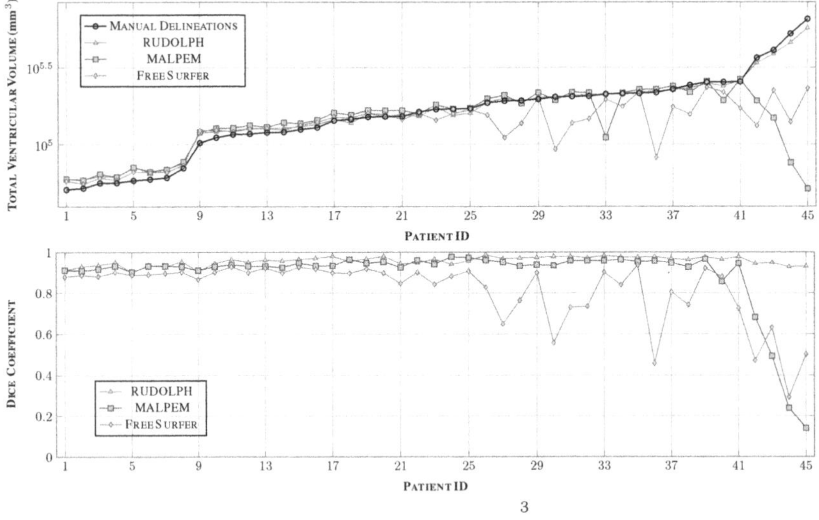

Fig. 2. The top row shows the mean volume in mm^3 for the manual masks and the three methods over the 45 NPH patients, ordered based on the volume of the manual masks. The y-axis uses a log scale to help differentiate the volumes of the different methods across the whole range of volumes. The bottom row shows the Dice coefficient over the same 45 NPH patients with the same ordering. The NPH patient shown in the top row of Fig. 1 has Patient ID #39 and the bottom row corresponds to Patient ID #43.

We processed the 45 NPH patients using RUDOLPH and two state-of-the-art whole brain segmentation methods: FreeSurfer (Version 5.3.0) [8] and MALPEM [9]. We ran FreeSurfer with the `-bigventricles` flag. We used an in-house [3,4] approach to skull strip the data, as we have found that this improves the performance of both FreeSurfer and MALPEM on our NPH cohort. The volumes generated by FreeSurfer, MALPEM, and RUDOLPH for the entire ventricular system are shown in the top row of Fig. 2; the patients are ordered based on the volume of the manual delineations which is also shown in the figure. The NPH patient shown in the top row of Fig. 1 corresponds to Patient ID #39 in Fig. 2, the bottom row of Fig. 1 corresponds to Patient ID #43. We computed the Dice coefficient [6] for these 45 NPH patients on the entire ventricle system, the results are reported in Table 1. A paired two-sided Wilcoxon Signed-Rank Test [16], without a correction for multiple comparisons, comparing FreeSurfer to MALPEM on the entire ventricle system yielded significant differences with a p-value <0.001. We also obtained a similar p-value (<0.001) when comparing MALPEM to RUDOLPH on the entire ventricle system. These Dice coefficients are shown in the bottom row of Fig. 2, ordered by the volume of the manual masks. We also computed the Dice coefficient for each of the automatically labeled ventricular cavities with the corresponding manual delineation; see Table 1 and Fig. 3. RUDOLPH produces more accurate segmentation of the third ventricle and the left and right lateral ventricles than both MALPEM and FreeSurfer; these results also reach statistical significance. The fourth ventricle is most accurately segmented by MALPEM, however it is not statistically significantly better than RUDOLPH (see Table 2).

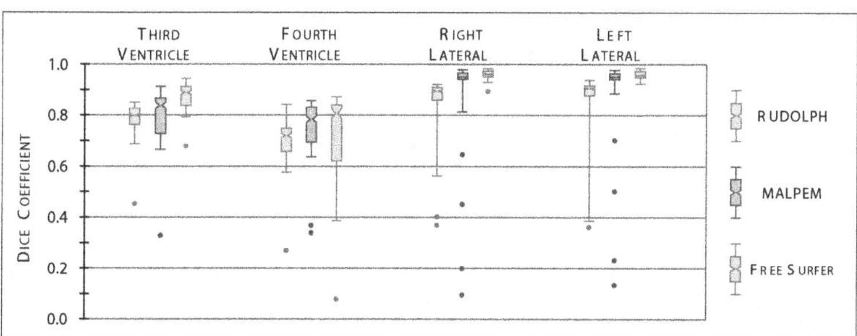

Fig. 3. Box plots of the Dice coefficient with respect to our manual masks over 18 NPH patients comparing the automatically generated labels from the three methods for four ventricular cavities: third ventricle, fourth ventricle, right lateral ventricle, and left lateral ventricle.

Table 1. The mean Dice coefficient (and standard deviation) over our population of NPH patients measuring similarity between manual labels and automatically generated labels from the three methods. For 45 NPH patients we compare the entire (Entire) ventricle system. For 18 of those 45 we compare four ventricular cavities, third ventricle (3rd), fourth ventricle (4th), right lateral ventricle (RLV), and left lateral ventricle (LLV).

	FreeSurfer	MALPEM	RUDOLPH
Entire	0.815 ($\pm$0.150)	0.890 ($\pm$0.172)	0.957 ($\pm$0.021)
3rd	0.775 ($\pm$0.091)	0.780 ($\pm$0.140)	0.869 ($\pm$0.065)
4th	0.656 ($\pm$0.156)	0.720 ($\pm$0.152)	0.694 ($\pm$0.205)
RLV	0.799 ($\pm$0.181)	0.810 ($\pm$0.278)	0.956 ($\pm$0.022)
LLV	0.803 ($\pm$0.192)	0.825 ($\pm$0.262)	0.959 ($\pm$0.018)

Table 2. p-values for a paired two-sided Wilcoxon Signed-Rank Test [16], without a correction for multiple comparisons, between the two methods listed for the noted ventricle cavity. This is across the 18 patients that are also compared to manual masks and presented in Fig. 3. The key for the ventricular cavities is: third ventricle – 3rd; fourth ventricle – 4th; right lateral ventricle – RLV; and left lateral ventricle – LLV.

Comparison	3rd	4th	RLV	LLV
FreeSurfer vs. MALPEM	0.6397	0.0007	0.2837	0.0987
FreeSurfer vs. RUDOLPH	0.0007	0.1187	0.0000	0.0000
MALPEM vs. RUDOLPH	0.0007	0.2462	0.0023	0.0016

4 Discussion and Conclusions

We have presented a method for whole brain segmentation that provides a robust segmentation of the ventricular system in patients with severely enlarged ventricles. We have shown that the approach is more robust on the ventricles than either FreeSurfer or MALPEM across 45 NPH patients; it consistently tracks the volume generated by the manual delineation of the ventricles better than either method as shown in the top row of Fig. 2. In particular, we note that both the FreeSurfer and MALPEM estimates of the ventricular CSF volume become more erratic as the volume increases. This is particularly troubling as the ventricles do naturally increase in size through natural brain atrophy over the time course of healthy patients. This study would call into question the validity of using these methods in a fully automated fashion without some quality assurance review of the results. We also note that FreeSurfer appears to level off and be unable to provide ventricular volumes above a certain level, which may be a limitation of the approach. MALPEM also exhibits instability in its results as the ventricular volume increases (see Fig. 2), however these do not always seem to be tied to the volume of the ventricles. As noted earlier the MALPEM estimates of the ventricular volume for Patient ID #39 are reasonable. Yet Patient ID #40 has a similar volume to Patient ID #39 and MALPEM performs poorly; whereas Patient ID #36 has less volume and MALPEM essentially fails. The results suggest that these patients may have significantly differently shaped structures which is leading to the failure of MALPEM. Our initial review of these results suggest that misregistrations within the multi-atlas phase of MALPEM may be the cause of these problems; which reinforces our belief that our enhancements to MALPEM are appropriate fixes for pathology cases. We also demonstrated that our approach can more accurately estimate the ventricular cavities of the lateral ventricles and the third ventricle (see Table 1).

Future work includes creating manual delineations on a larger cohort of patients—in particular patients suffering from ventriculomegaly by other causes. We also plan to further refine the parcellation of the ventricles to include the subchambers—anterior, occipital, and temporal horns of the lateral ventricles. A future goal will be correlating the volumetrics of these structures with surgical outcomes for NPH patients.

Acknowledgments. This work was supported by the NIH/NINDS under grant R21-NS096497. Support was also provided by the National Multiple Sclerosis Society grant RG-1507-05243 and the Dept. of Defense Center for Neuroscience and Regenerative Medicine.

References

1. Adams, R.D., et al.: Symptomatic occult hydrocephalus with normal cerebrospinal-fluid pressure - a treatable syndrome. New Eng. J. Med. **273**(3), 117–126 (1965)
2. Avants, B.B., et al.: Symmetric diffeomorphic image registration with cross-correlation: evaluating automated labeling of elderly and neurodegenerative brain. Med. Image Anal. **12**(1), 26–41 (2008)
3. Carass, A., et al.: A joint registration and segmentation approach to skull stripping. In: 4th International Symposium on Biomedical Imaging (ISBI 2007), pp. 656–659. IEEE (2007)
4. Carass, A., et al.: Simple paradigm for extra-cerebral tissue removal: algorithm and analysis. NeuroImage **56**(4), 1982–1992 (2010)
5. Coupe, P., et al.: Patch-based segmentation using expert priors: application to hippocampus and ventricle segmentation. NeuroImage **54**, 940–954 (2011)
6. Dice, L.R.: Measures of the amount of ecologic association between species. Ecology **26**(3), 297–302 (1945)
7. Ellingsen, L.M., et al.: Segmentation and labeling of the ventricular system in normal pressure hydrocephalus using patch-based tissue classification and multi-atlas labeling. In: Proceedings of SPIE Medical Imaging (SPIE-MI 2016), San Diego, CA, vol. 9784, p. 97840G–97840G-7, 27 February–3 March 2016 (2016)
8. Fischl, B.: FreeSurfer. NeuroImage **62**(2), 774–781 (2012)
9. Ledig, C., et al.: Robust whole-brain segmentation: application to traumatic brain injury. Med. Image Anal. **21**, 40–58 (2015)
10. Poca, M.A., et al.: Is the placement of shunts in patients with idiopathic normal pressure hydrocephalus worth the risk? Results of a study based on continuous monitoring of intracranial pressure. J. Neurosurg. **100**(5), 855–866 (2004)

11. Roy, S., Carass, A., Prince, J.L., Pham, D.L.: Subject specific sparse dictionary learning for atlas based brain MRI segmentation. In: Wu, G., Zhang, D., Zhou, L. (eds.) MLMI 2014. LNCS, vol. 8679, pp. 248–255. Springer, Cham (2014). doi:10.1007/978-3-319-10581-9_31
12. Roy, S., et al.: Subject-specific sparse dictionary learning for atlas-based brain MRI segmentation. IEEE J. Biomed. Health Inform. **19**(5), 1598–1609 (2015)
13. Shiee, N., Bazin, P.-L., Cuzzocreo, J.L., Blitz, A., Pham, D.L.: Segmentation of brain images using adaptive atlases with application to ventriculomegaly. In: Székely, G., Hahn, H.K. (eds.) IPMI 2011. LNCS, vol. 6801, pp. 1–12. Springer, Heidelberg (2011). doi:10.1007/978-3-642-22092-0_1
14. Toma, A.K., et al.: Systematic review of the outcome of shunt surgery in idiopathic normal-pressure hydrocephalus. Acta Neurochir. **155**, 1977–1980 (2013)
15. Van Leemput, K., et al.: Automated model-based tissue classification of MR images of the brain. IEEE Trans. Med. Imaging **18**, 897–908 (1999)
16. Wilcoxon, F.: Individual comparisons by ranking methods. Biom. Bull. **1**(6), 80–83 (1945)
17. Zhang, J.: The mean field theory in EM procedures for Markov random fields. IEEE Trans. Signal Process. **40**, 2570–2583 (1992)

Hippocampus Subfield Segmentation Using a Patch-Based Boosted Ensemble of Autocontext Neural Networks

José V. Manjón[1(✉)] and Pierrick Coupe[2,3]

[1] Instituto de Aplicaciones de Las Tecnologías de La Información Y de Las Comunicaciones Avanzadas (ITACA), Universitat Politècnica de València, Camino de Vera s/n, 46022 Valencia, Spain
jmanjon@fis.upv.es
[2] Univ. Bordeaux, LaBRI, UMR 5800, PICTURA, 33400 Talence, France
[3] CNRS, LaBRI, UMR 5800, PICTURA, 33400 Talence, France

Abstract. The hippocampus is a brain structure that is involved in several cognitive functions such as memory and learning. It is a structure of great interest in the study of the healthy and diseased brain due to its relationship to several neurodegenerative pathologies. In this work, we propose a novel patch-based method that uses an ensemble of boosted neural networks to perform the hippocampus subfield segmentation on multimodal MRI. This new method minimizes both random and systematic errors using an overcomplete autocontext patch-based labeling using a novel boosting strategy. The proposed method works well on high resolution MRI but also on standard resolution images after superresolution. Finally, the proposed method was compared with a similar state-of-the-art methods showing better results in terms of both accuracy and efficiency.

1 Introduction

The hippocampus (HC) is a complex gray matter structure located under the surface of each temporal lobe. It is involved in many cognitive functions such as memory and spatial reasoning [1]. It has been largely studied in the last years to understand its healthy evolution across the lifespan in normal aging [2] but also due to its key role in several dysfunctions such as epilepsy [3], schizophrenia [4] or Alzheimer's disease [5].

The hippocampus is composed of multiple subfields that can be divided into sections called the dentate gyrus, the cornu ammonis (CA) and the subiculum. The CA is also subdivided in sub-sections CA1, CA2, CA3, CA4, layers alveus, stratum oriens, stratum pyramidale, stratum radiatum, stratum lancosum and stratum moleculare. These layers present a high neuron density and are very compact so high resolution imaging is required to identify them.

Due to this morphological complexity and MR related image resolution limitations, mainly whole hippocampus volume analysis has been performed in the past by segmenting it as a single object [6]. Even with this limitations whole HC volume has been shown to be a good biomarker for Alzheimer's disease [7]. However, hippocampus

© Springer International Publishing AG 2017
G. Wu et al. (Eds.): Patch-MI 2017, LNCS 10530, pp. 29–36, 2017.
DOI: 10.1007/978-3-319-67434-6_4

subfields have shown to be affected differently by AD and normal aging in ex-vivo studies [5] which makes them excellent candidates for early diagnosis.

Although high resolution MRI is becoming more accessible in research scenarios, manual segmentation, which is the most accurate analysis method, is not a feasible option since it is a highly time consuming procedure which requires expert trained raters taking many hours per case.

To overcome this problem some automated segmentation solutions have been developed in the last years. One of the first methods was proposed by Van Leemput et al. using a statistical model of MR image formation around the hippocampus to produce automatic segmentation [7]. Recently, Iglesias et al. pursued this work and replaced the model by a more accurate atlas generated using ultra-high resolution ex-vivo MR images [8]. Chakravarty et al. proposed a multiatlas method based on the estimation of several non-linear deformations and a label fusion step [9]. Also using a multiatlas approach, Yushkevich proposed a method where a multiatlas approach is combined with a similarity-weighted voting and a learning-based label bias correction [10] and Romero et al. also proposed a multiatlas multispectral method [21].

In this work, we propose a fast and accurate patch-based method to segment the hippocampus subfields using an ensemble of boosted neural networks. In the next sections, we will describe the method details as well as some experiments to demonstrate the accuracy and efficiency of the proposed approach.

2 Materials and Methods

2.1 Image Data

In this paper, we used a High Resolution (HR) dataset composed of 25 cases with T1-weighted and T2-weighted images to construct a library of manually labeled cases. This dataset includes 25 subjects from a public repository (http://www.nitrc.org/projects/mni-hisub25) (31 ± 7 yrs, 12 males, 13 females) with manually-drawn labels dividing the HC in three parts (CA1-3, DG-CA4 and Subiculum). MRI data from each subject consist of an isotropic 3D-MPRAGE T1-weighted ($0.6 \times 0.6 \times 0.6$ mm^3) and anisotropic 2D T2-weighted TSE images ($0.4 \times 0.4 \times 2$ mm^3). Images underwent automated correction for intensity non-uniformity, intensity standardization and were linearly registered to the MNI152 space. T1w and T2w images were resampled to a resolution of 0.4 mm^3 (Fig. 1). To reduce interpolation artifacts, the T2w data was upsampled using a non-local super resolution method [19]. For more details about the labeling protocol see the original paper [11].

2.2 Preprocessing

All the images (T1 and T2) were first filtered with a spatially adaptive non-local means filter [15] and inhomogeneity corrected using the N4 method [16]. Later, they were linearly registered to the Montreal Neurological Institute space (MNI) using the ANTS package [17] and the MNI152 template. Next, we left-right flipped the images and cropped them to the right hippocampus area to produce 50 right hippocampus crops.

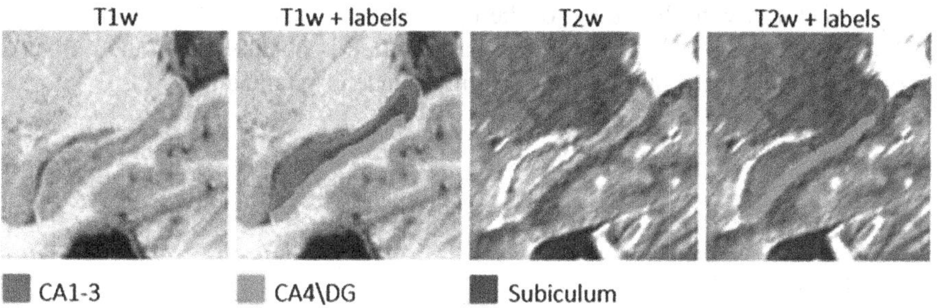

Fig. 1. Example of an HR MRI case. Figure shows T1w and T2w images and its corresponding manual segmentation.

After that, we non-linearly registered the cropped images to the cropped MNI152 template to better match the hippocampus anatomy. Finally, we normalized the image intensities using Nyúl and Udupa [18] method. Hippocampus labels were spatially registered to the same space.

2.3 Proposed Method

After the described preprocessing, a region of interest (ROI) is computed fusing all manual segmentations of the library and dilating the resulting region with a $5 \times 5 \times 5$ voxels kernel to create a HC candidate region. For each voxel of this candidate region a feature set is created to be used to train a classifier. Several classifiers can be used to relate the image features and the corresponding labels. Lately high performance classifiers such as random forest [12] have been used. In our proposed method, we have used a neural network-based classifier [13].

- ***Features***: The features used to train the network were three 3D patches per image modality of different size around the voxel/s to be classified, the x, y and z voxel coordinates of the center voxel of the patches and a value representing the *a priori* label probability. This apriori label probability map was obtained computing the average of all training label masks (convolved with a 5 mm^3 Gaussian kernel). In our experiments, we used a P_1 of size $3 \times 3 \times 3$, a P_2 of $7 \times 7 \times 7$ and P_3 of $9 \times 9 \times 9$ voxels (however, for efficiency, we subsampled the patches P_2 and P_3 so we took only 27 samples uniformly spaced in all three dimensions). This leads to a feature vector X of 166 elements (i.e. 27 for P_1, 27 for P_2 and 27 for P_3 on T1, the same for T2, x, y and z coordinates and the prior probability).
- ***Network topology***: A feedforward multilayer perceptron with two hidden layers was used. The network that we used had $166 \times 85 \times 55 \times 27$ weights. The network output is a patch of the same size of P_1. Note that an overcomplete approach was used so each voxel has contributions from several adjacent patches. This improves segmentation accuracy (more votes per voxel) and enforces the final label regularity. To further improve classification results a second autocontext network is trained using an expanded feature vector constructed concatenating the original

feature vector X with the output of the first network. This leads to a feature vector X_a of 193 elements (166 + 27). Final classification is obtained from the output of network 2. Note that both networks are independently trained (Fig. 2).

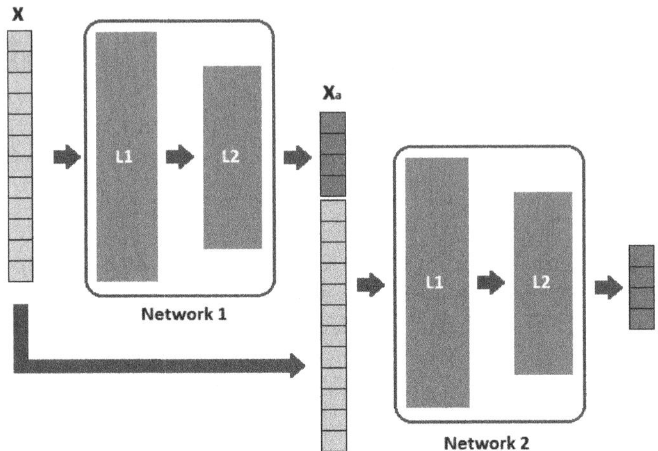

Fig. 2. Autocontext neural network. Original feature vector x used to train network 1 is expanded using the output of the network (posterior probabilities) to train network 2.

Ensemble-Based Classification

A common approach for improving classification results is the use of the so-called ensemble learning. Ensemble methods (i.e. combination of several classifiers) allow in general to improve classification results by minimizing random and systematic errors.

In our proposed method, we have used a boosting strategy to leverage classification accuracy. Boosting [14] is an algorithm that combines the output of several classifiers to minimize the variance and bias of the final classification. In boosting, each classifier is trained using the information of the previous one to minimize the errors of the current prediction. This is done giving more weight to the samples wrongly classified by the previous classifier or performing a non-random selection on the training dataset selecting with higher probability samples wrongly classified previously. While typically each network uses random initial weights (network reset) we decided to use the weights of the previous network as done in transfer learning which improves ensemble classifier accuracy while minimizing training time due to faster convergence. Finally, the different classifier outputs are combined according to their accuracy.

We trained four ensembles of M autocontext modules (Fig. 2) (one ensemble per subfield plus the background) over the whole hippocampus region and each voxel was labeled with the class of higher network output.

3 Experiments and Results

In this section, a set of experiments are presented to show the performance of the proposed method. All the experiments have been done by processing the cases from the described library splitting the 50 cases first into a 30 training cases set and 20 test cases and later switching training and test datasets to evaluate the whole dataset.

3.1 Ensemble Training

We explored two variants of ensemble training, the classical one with network reset and one without reset. For these experiments, we trained M = 10 autocontext networks using only 10000 samples randomly selected from the candidate regions of the training dataset. All resulting networks outputs were averaged according to the accuracy to produce the final output.

We evaluated the impact of the two boosting variants (with and without reset) and estimated the optimal number of neural networks. In Fig. 3 (left), the evolution of the DICE coefficient (during training without reset) as a function of the number of individual and averaged trained networks is shown. In Fig. 3 (right), the same results with reset option are also shown.

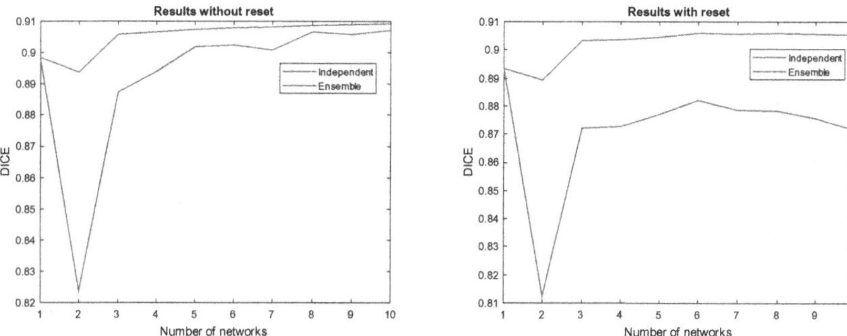

Fig. 3. Left: Dice coefficient in function of the number of networks for each network in nthe ensemble and for the ensemble prediction with the proposed boosting. Right: Same results with classical boosting. Note that using previous network in the embeding not only improves overall ensemble accuarcy but also produces more accurate individual networks.

As can be noticed, both boosting variants improved the classification results reaching a plateau at around 10 networks. However, no-reset boosting produced a more pronounced improvement compared to classical reset approach (0.9091 versus 0.9052). To understand the improved results we can look at the accuracy of each individual network of the ensemble. As can be noticed, reseted networks show a pseudo stable behaviour while non-reseted networks show maintained improvements as long as the number of ensemble networks increases. In fact, non-reseted last individual networks almost reach the accuracy of the whole ensemble.

With this settings, we trained the final network ensemble (M = 10) using randomly selected sets of 1000000 samples from the total population of 2600000 patches. To train the 4 ensembles took around 8 h while the time to segment a new case is around 10 s. To evaluate all 50 cases we trained two ensemble sets (one using the 30 training cases and applied to the remaining 20 cases and another trained on the 20 cases and applied to the 30 cases). We could do a leave-one-out approach to further improving the results but this would result on a large training time of around two weeks. Table 1 shows the dice coefficient of the different subfields for the 50 cases. We have also included the results when using only the best network instead of the ensemble (thus requiring only 1 s to perform the segmentation).

Table 1. Mean DICE and standard deviation for each structure segmentation using two variants of the proposed method. Best results in bold.

Structure	Proposed (best network)	Proposed (ensemble)
Average	0.8681	**0.8695**
CA1-3	0.8992	**0.9001**
CA4\DG	0.8384	**0.8404**
Subiculum	0.8667	**0.8678**
Hippocampus	0.9518	**0.9523**

3.2 Standard Resolution vs High Resolution

High resolution MR images are not widely available, especially in clinical environments. For this reason, we analyzed the effectiveness of the proposed method on upsampled standard resolution images. For this purpose, we reduced the resolution of the library HR images by a factor 2 by convolving the HR images with a $2 \times 2 \times 2$ boxcar kernel and then decimating the resulting image. The down-sampled images were upsampled by a factor 2 using BSpline interpolation and a superresolution method called Local Adaptive SR (LASR) [19]. Results are shown in Table 2. As can be noticed, segmentations performed on images upsampled with SR were better than using BSpline interpolation. Moreover, this experiment shows that the proposed method is able to produce competitive results even when using standard resolution images.

Table 2. Mean DICE for each structure segmentation using the high resolution library and applying BSpline interpolation and LASR to the previously downsampled image to be segmented. Best results in bold.

Structure	BSpline	LASR	HR
Average	0.8595	0.8662	**0.8695**
CA1-3	0.8930	0.8981	**0.9001**
CA4\DG	0.8250	0.8349	**0.8404**
Subiculum	0.8605	0.8655	**0.8678**
Hippocampus	0.9480	0.9513	**0.9523**

3.3 Comparison

We compared our method with other recent methods applied to hippocampus segmentation using the same number of structures and labeling protocol. The compared methods are called ASHS [10] and Surfpatch [20]. Table 3 shows that the proposed method obtained higher DICE coefficients for all the structures. In terms of computation efficiency, our method requires only few seconds while ASHS and Surfpatch have an execution time of several hours per case.

Table 3. Mean DICE in the native space for each structure. Segmentation performed by ASHS, SurfPatch, proposed method and human rater (intra-rater and inter-rater). Best results (for automatic segmentation) in bold.

Structure	ASHS	SurfPatch	Proposed	Inter-rater	Intra-rater
Average	0.8513	0.8503	**0.8584**	0.8833	0.9113
CA1-3	0.8736	0.8743	**0.8903**	0.8760	0.9290
CA4\DG	0.8254	0.8271	**0.8283**	0.9030	0.9000
Subiculum	0.8548	0.8495	**0.8565**	0.8710	0.9050

4 Discussion

In this paper, we present a new hippocampus subfield segmentation method based on a boosted ensemble of autocontext neural networks. The proposed method achieves state-of-the-art accuracy very efficiently. Furthermore, the proposed method has been shown to perform well on standard resolution images, obtaining competitive results on typical clinical data. This fact is very important because it will allow analyzing large amounts of legacy data. Finally, it has been also shown that the proposed method compares well to another related state-of-art method obtaining better results in terms of both accuracy and reduced execution time.

Acknowledgements. This research was supported by the Spanish UPV2016-0099 grant from Universitat Politécnica de Valencia. This study has been also carried out with financial support from the French State, managed by the French National Research Agency (ANR) in the frame of the Investments for the future Program IdEx Bordeaux (ANR-10-IDEX-03-02, HL-MRI Project) and Cluster of excellence CPU and TRAIL (HR-DTI ANR-10-LABX-57).

References

1. Milner, B.: Psychological defects produced by temporal lobe excision. Res. Publ. Assoc. Res. Nerv. Ment. Dis. **36**, 244–257 (1958)
2. Petersen, R., et al.: Memory and MRI-based hippocampal volumes in aging and AD. Neurology **54**(3), 581–587 (2000)
3. Cendes, F., et al.: MRI volumetric measurement of amygdala and hippocampus in temporal lobe epilepsy. Neurology **43**(4), 719–725 (1993)

4. Altshuler, L.L., et al.: Amygdala enlargement *in bipo*lar disorder and hippocampal reduction in schizophrenia: an MRI study demonstrating neuroanatomic specificity Arch. Gen. Psychiatry **55**(7), 663 (1998)
5. Braak, H., Braak, E.: Neuropathological stageing of Alzheimer-related changes. Acta Neuropathol. **82**(4), 239–259 (1991)
6. Chupin, M., et al.: Fully automatic hippocampus segmentation and classification in Alzheimer's disease and mild cognitive impairment applied on data from ADNI. Hippocampus **19**(6), 579–587 (2009)
7. Van Leemput, K., et al.: Automated segmentation of hippocampal subfields from ultra-high resolution in vivo MRI. Hippocampus **19**(6), 549–557 (2009)
8. Iglesias, J.E., et al.: A computational atlas of the hippocampal formation using ex vivo, ultra-high resolution MRI: application to adaptive segmentation of in vivo MRI. NeuroImage **115**(15), 117–137 (2015)
9. Chakravarty, M., et al.: Performing label-fusion-based segmentation using multiple automatically generated templates. Hum. Brain Mapp. **10**(34), 2635–2654 (2013)
10. Yushkevich, P.A., et al.: Automated volumetry and regional thickness analysis of hippocampal subfields and medial temporal cortical structures in mild cognitive impairment. Hum. Brain Mapp. **36**(1), 258–287 (2015)
11. Kulaga-Yoskovitz, J., Bernhardt, B.C., Hong, S., Mansi, T., Liang, K.E., van der Kouwe, A. J.W., Smallwood, J., Bernasconi, A., Bernasconi, N.: Multi-contrast submillimetric 3Tesla hippocampal subfield segmentation protocol and dataset. Sci Data **2**, 150059 (2015)
12. Serag, A., et al.: SEGMA: an automatic SEGMentation approach for human brain MRI using sliding window and random forests. Front Neuroinform. **11**, 2 (2017)
13. Manjón, J.V., et al.: HIST: hyperintensity segmentation tool. In: PatchMI workshop, MICCAI2016, Athens (2016)
14. Schapire, R.E.: The strength of weak learnability. Mach. Learn. **5**(2), 197–227 (1990)
15. Manjón, J.V., et al.: Adaptive non-local means denoising of MR images with spatially varying noise levels. J Magn. Reson. Imaging **31**, 192–203 (2010)
16. Tustison, N.J., et al.: N4ITK: improved N3 bias correction. IEEE Trans. Med. Imaging **29** (6), 1310–1320 (2010)
17. Avants, B.B., et al.: Advanced normalization tools (ANTS). Insight J. (2009)
18. Nyúl, L.G., Udupa, J.K.: On standardizing the MR image intensity scale. Magn. Reson. Med. **42**(6), 1072–1081 (1999)
19. Coupé, P., et al.: Collaborative patch-based super-resolution for diffusion-weighted images. NeuroImage **83**, 245–261 (2013)
20. Caldairou, B., Bernhardt, B.C., Kulaga-Yoskovitz, J., Kim, H., Bernasconi, N., Bernasconi, A.: A surface patch-based segmentation method for hippocampal subfields. In: Ourselin, S., Joskowicz, L., Sabuncu, M.R., Unal, G., Wells, W. (eds.) MICCAI 2016 Part II. LNCS, vol. 9901, pp. 379–387. Springer, Cham (2016). doi:10.1007/978-3-319-46723-8_44
21. Romero, J.E., Coupe, P., Manjón, J.V.: High resolution hippocampus subfield segmentation using multispectral multiatlas patch-based label fusion. In: Wu, G., Coupé, P., Zhan, Y., Munsell, B.C., Rueckert, D. (eds.) Patch-MI 2016. LNCS, vol. 9993, pp. 117–124. Springer, Cham (2016). doi:10.1007/978-3-319-47118-1_15

On the Role of Patch Spaces in Patch-Based Label Fusion

Oualid M. Benkarim[1(✉)], Gemma Piella[1], Miguel Angel González Ballester[1,2], and Gerard Sanroma[1]

[1] Universitat Pompeu Fabra, Barcelona, Spain
oualid.benkarim@upf.edu
[2] ICREA, Barcelona, Spain

Abstract. Multi-atlas segmentation has shown promising results in the segmentation of biomedical images. In the most common approach, registration is used to warp the atlases to the target space and then the warped atlas labelmaps are fused into a consensus segmentation. Label fusion in target space has shown to produce very accurate segmentations although at the expense of registering all atlases to each target image. Moreover, appearance and label information used by label fusion is extracted from the warped atlases, which are subject to interpolation errors. This work explores the role of extracting this information from the native spaces and adapt two label fusion approaches to this scheme. Results on the segmentation of subcortical brain structures indicate that using atlases in their native space yields superior performance than warping the atlases to the target. Moreover, using the native space lessens the computational requirements in terms of number of registrations and learning.

Keywords: Label fusion · MRI · Multiatlas segmentation · Patch space

1 Introduction

Multi-atlas segmentation (MAS) has recently shown promising results in the segmentation of biomedical images. In the MAS setting, multiple atlases are used to segment a given target image, as opposed to single atlas-based segmentation, where there is only one atlas. By using multiple atlases, MAS can better capture the anatomical variability of the entire population. The major steps common to all MAS approaches consist on registration and label fusion (LF). During registration, the atlases and the target image are spatially transformed to the same space in order to establish spatial correspondences. Then, LF finds the optimal strategy to combine all atlas labelmaps into a consensus segmentation on the target image. The present work focuses on patch-based LF [4], which uses a 3D patch around the voxel of interest to represent its appearance information. There are several choices in patch-based LF that need to be considered in the fusion process: fusion strategy, fusion space and patch space.

© Springer International Publishing AG 2017
G. Wu et al. (Eds.): Patch-MI 2017, LNCS 10530, pp. 37–44, 2017.
DOI: 10.1007/978-3-319-67434-6_5

Fusion Strategy. The strategy used to fuse the multiple atlas labelmaps is an important step in MAS. In this work, we focus on two widely-known strategies. Given a set of atlas patches x_i and their corresponding labels y_i, the target patch x_t is segmented as follows:

1. Similarity-based LF: atlas labels, y_i, are weighted according to the similarity of their intensity patches with the target patch [4,6]. The more similar x_i is to the target patch x_t, the higher the contribution of its label, y_i.
2. Learning-based LF: these approaches learn from the atlas patches x_i a function that maps local image appearances to the corresponding label, y_i [3,5]. When a target image arrives, this function is used to predict a label for each target voxel.

Fusion Space. This is the space where the estimated segmentation is computed via LF. It is typically done in one of the following spaces:

1. Target fusion space: the target labelmap is computed directly in the target space. To that end, spatial transformations between the atlases and the target image are computed to warp the atlases to the target space, where LF takes place (see Fig. 1).
2. Template fusion space: the target labelmap is computed in a template space. To that end, both atlases and target are warped to a template space (e.g., MNI152) and LF is performed in this common space using warped atlases $\tilde{A}_i$ and the warped target $\tilde{T}$. The estimated segmentation is then warped back to the target space (see Fig. 2).

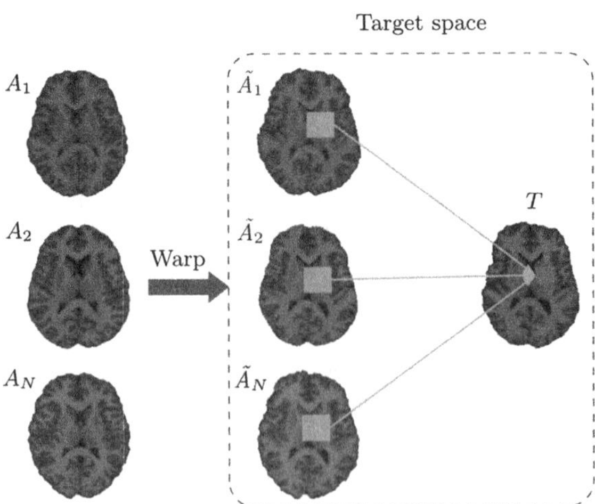

Fig. 1. Target fusion space. The target labelmap is computed directly in the target space via LF using the warped atlases $\tilde{A}_i$. (Color figure online)

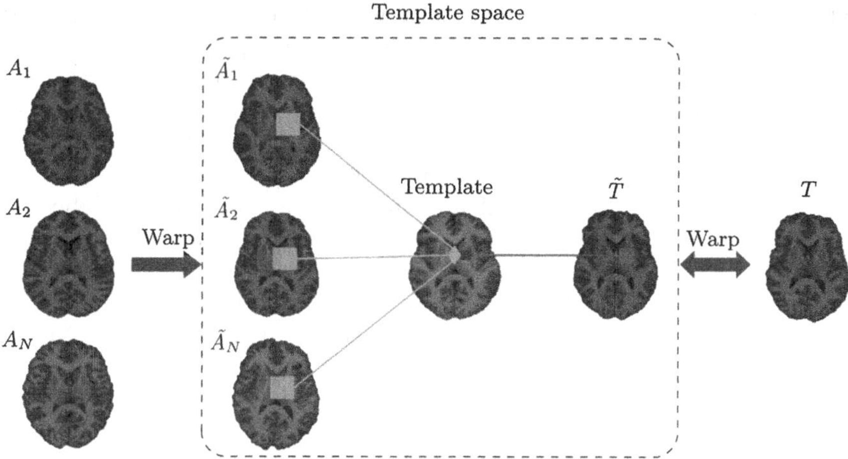

Fig. 2. Template fusion space: target labelmap is computed in the template space using the warped atlases and target to the template space. Then, the estimated segmentation is warped back to the target space.

In the vast literature on MAS, the most common space used to perform LF is the target space (i.e., target fusion space), especially for methods using similarity-based fusion strategies. The main advantage of target fusion space is that the target labelmap does not need to be warped back to the target space, thus incurring in label interpolation errors. Also, the target image suffers no distortion due to registration-based interpolations. However, given N training atlases, the computational burden of this approach is high because it requires N registrations per target image. In this direction, researchers proposed non-local patch-based label fusion strategies that only use coarse registrations to lower the computational requirements [4,6]. Although the computational burden can be alleviated by composing the atlas-to-target registration through a template.

The template fusion space is usually adopted by methods using a learning-based fusion strategy [7], since classifiers to label each voxel can be trained offline. On the other hand, using the target fusion space implies learning the classifiers online for each new target image, which is computationally demanding [5,8]. Classifiers are trained on the warped atlases to segment a single target image and cannot be reused to segment other target images. Here, atlas selection [1] can be used to reduce the size of the training set and hence learning times, though atlas selection introduces another free parameter (i.e., the number of most similar atlases) into the MAS setting, to be chosen during an intermediate validation step, for instance.

Patch Space. Patch space refers to the spaces used to extract the appearance (e.g. patches) and label information used in LF. In most approaches, the patch space coincides with the fusion space. Particularly, LF in target fusion space is based on patches extracted from the atlases warped to the target, $\tilde{A}_i$ (see green arrows in Fig. 1), not the atlases in their native space (i.e., A_i). Similarly, in template fusion space, patches are extracted from the atlases and the target image warped to the template (i.e., $\tilde{A}_i$ and $\tilde{T}$ respectively, as shown in Fig. 2). Irrespective of fusion space, the warped atlases are subject to interpolation errors. This is an important drawback because the interpolation strategy used for the atlas intensity images (e.g., linear) is different from the one used for the labelmaps (e.g., nearest neighbors). In this way, a deformed labelmap might be no longer faithful to its corresponding deformed intensity image under the manual segmentation protocol followed by the expert. In case of using the template as fusion space, there is an additional source of error due to interpolation of the estimated labelmap, which occurs when warping it back to the target space.

Little attention is paid by researchers in MAS to the space where the patches are extracted from. In this work, we propose a LF approach that uses appearance and label information from the native spaces of both atlases and target images, the so-called *native patch space*. Thus, registration is used to only find spatial correspondences between the atlases and the target image, without deforming any of them. The advantages of native patch space are threefold: (1) there is no need to warp the atlases, thus avoiding any inaccuracies between atlas images and corresponding labelmaps due to interpolation artifacts. This allows LF to be driven by the true appearance patterns used by the expert to create the ground truth, (2) avoiding warping the atlases also implies a higher storage efficiency, since there is no need to keep two instances of each atlas (i.e., the original and the warped one), (3) learning-based fusion strategies can be applied directly in the target fusion space, whithout the need to train the classifiers online for each target.

The paper is organized as follows. In Sect. 2 we present the details of our method. In Sect. 3 we describe the experimental setting and present the results, and in Sect. 4 we conclude the paper.

2 Method

The proposed approach is based on the observation that LF in template or target fusion spaces relies on different (i.e., deformed) versions of the atlases and not the original ones, and therefore, there exists a risk of introducing noise in the segmentation process due to interpolation errors. On the contrary, in our approach, the mappings computed during registration are only used to find spatial correspondences between the atlases and the target image, but the images are not deformed. In order to avoid registering the atlases each time a novel target image arrives, atlases are registered to a common reference space. Figure 3 illustrates how LF is carried out in our novel approach. Throughout the rest of the paper, we will refer to it as LF in native patch space.

In the proposed approach, we adopt a non-local patch-based approach [4]. Let ϕ_i be the mapping of the i-th atlas, A_i, to the template space and ϕ_t the mapping of the target image. For each voxel v_t and corresponding patch x_t (see red box in Fig. 3) on the target image:

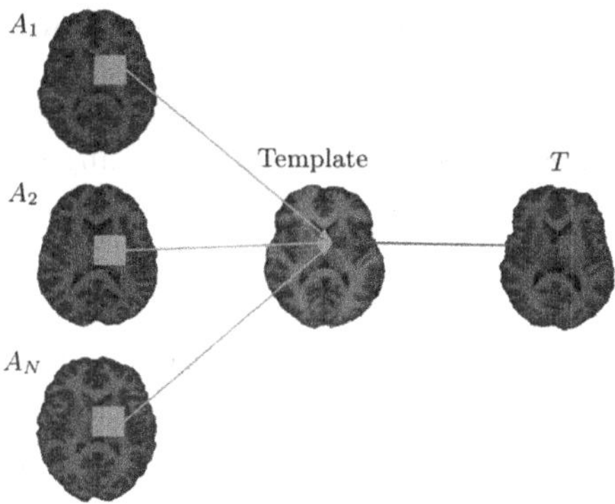

Fig. 3. LF in native patch space. Correspondences between the atlases A_i and the target image T are used to extract the patches from their respective native spaces. Target labelmaps are directly computed in the target fusion space.(Color figure online)

1. Find corresponding voxel in template space (red arrow in Fig. 3):
$$\tilde{v} = \phi_t(v_t). \tag{1}$$
2. Find corresponding voxels in each atlas space (green arrows in Fig. 3):
$$v_i = \phi_i^{-1}(\phi_t(v_t)) = \phi_i^{-1}(\tilde{v}),\ i = 1, \ldots, N. \tag{2}$$
with i indexing the atlases in the database.
3. Extract patches and corresponding labels in the neighborhood of v_i (see green boxes in Fig. 3):
$$D = \{(x_{ij}, y_{ij})|\forall j \in S(v_i),\ i = 1, \ldots, N\} \tag{3}$$
where $y_{ij} \in \{-1, +1\}$ is the label of the j-th voxel in the neighborhood of v_i, denoted as $S(v_i)$, indicating foreground (i.e., $+1$) or background (i.e., -1).
4. Label target patch x_t using the set of patches D and some LF strategy as explained in the following.

The first fusion strategy is a similarity-based approach (SimLF) [4]. The SimLF strategy estimates the target label as a weighted combination of atlas labels, where atlas patches more similar to the target patch have higher contribution. It is defined as follows:

$$\hat{y}_t = sign\Big(\sum_{k=1}^{|D|} K(x_k, x_t) y_k\Big) \tag{4}$$

where $K(\cdot, \cdot)$ is a similarity measure between patches, and $|\cdot|$ denotes cardinality. Here, we use the exponential of the negative SSD as similarity measurement [4], defined as $K(x_t, x_k) = \exp(-\|x_t - x_k\|^2/\gamma)$, where γ is a normalization constant defined as $\gamma = \min \|x_k - x_t\|_2$ [4].

The next fusion strategy (LearnLF) consists on learning a labeling function that relates the patch intensities and their corresponding anatomical labels (x_k, y_k) using as training set the atlas patches and labels in D. Learning-based fusion strategies have already been proposed [5,8]. Using the well-known kernel-SVM for training the labeling function, the expression for estimating the target labels at test time is defined as follows:

$$\hat{y}_t = sign(\sum_{k=1}^{|D|} K(x_k, x_t) y_k \alpha_k + b) \tag{5}$$

where $K(\cdot,\cdot)$ is the RBF kernel defined as $K = \exp(-\|x_t - x_k\|^2/\gamma)$, with γ being the kernel width hyperparameter of kernel-SVM, and α_k and b are the coefficients of the support vectors and the intercept, respectively, which are computed offline during training.

Similarly to SimLF, LearnLF also weighs the contribution of the altas labels based on their similarity. Note the striking similarity between SimLF and LearnLF when using the RBF kernel in LearnLF. Key differences between both approaches are that LearnLF includes the learned coefficients α_k which, by definition of kernel-SVM, are only different than zero for the atlas patches playing the role of so-called support vectors. This could be interpreted as a form of patch selection. Finally, note that due to the fact that the proposed approach uses the native patch space, the atlas training patches for each classifier are invariant to the to-be-labeled target image, and therefore the classifiers for each point can be learned offline.

3 Experiments

All methods were evaluated on the MICCAI 2013 SATA Challenge dataset[1]. This dataset is composed of 35 T1-w MR images of control subjects with ground-truth segmentations available for seven subcortical structures: accumbens, amygdala, caudate, hippocampus, pallidum, putamen and thalamus proper.

All images were registered to the MNI152 template. For label fusion in target fusion space, pairwise mappings between the images were obtained by composing the transformations through the template. Furthermore, for image intensity to be consistent across atlases, histogram matching was used.

We compared the LF performance using all the patch spaces, namely, template, target and the proposed native patch space. Both SimLF and LearnLF fusion strategies were used in each of the patch spaces. Different patch and neighborhood sizes were used, with a radius of 1 and 2. For validation, a 3-fold cross-validation procedure was used with Dice similarity coefficient to assess the performance. Finally, all experiments were repeated using 2 registration settings: affine and non-rigid using the symmetric diffeomorphic mapping of ANTs [2].

Figure 4 shows mean overall Dice scores achieved by the tested LF strategies for different registration settings, comparing their performance depending on

[1] https://masi.vuse.vanderbilt.edu/workshop2013.

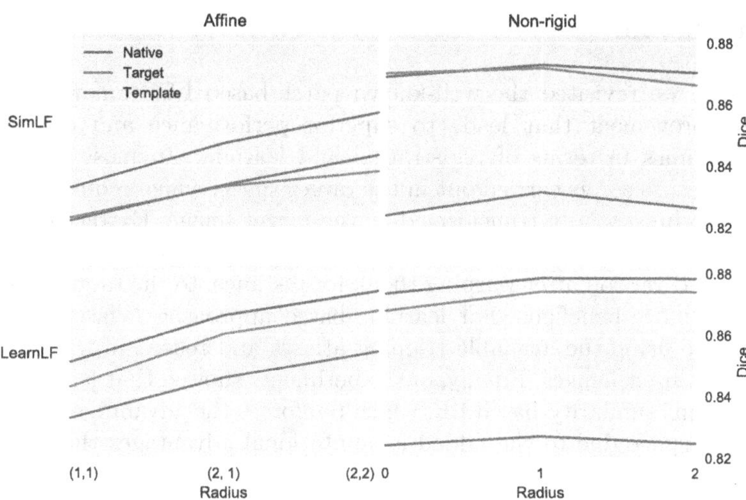

Fig. 4. Comparison of different patch spaces (colored lines), different fusion strategies and different registration settings. Top row: SimLF. Bottom row LearnLF. Left column: Affine registration. Right column: non-rigid registration. Vertical axis represents performance (Dice score) and horizontal axis indicate different patch and neighborhood radius values.(Color figure online)

patch space. Table 1 reports overall dice scores using a radius of 2 (i.e., size of $5 \times 5 \times 5$) for both patch and neighborhood search, with which all methods reached their best performance. Regardless of patch and neighborhood sizes, when using the native patch space, both SimLF and LearnLF produced the best segmentations. Moreover, for affine registration, the difference in performance when compared with LF in target space (i.e., target patch space) is the largest. Finally, it is worth noting that the LearnLF achieved better performance than SimLF, which highlights the importance of the learning approach versus the similarity-based approach.

Table 1. Overall performance in terms of average Dice overlap (and standard deviation) for the different patch spaces. Bold type indicates the best average segmentation performance.

	Affine		Non-rigid	
	SimLF	LearnLF	SimLF	LearnLF
Template	0.843 ± 0.040	0.855 ± 0.031	0.826 ± 0.036	0.825 ± 0.037
Target	0.838 ± 0.052	0.868 ± 0.032	0.866 ± 0.032	0.874 ± 0.027
Native	$\mathbf{0.857 \pm 0.044}$	$\mathbf{0.874 \pm 0.030}$	$\mathbf{0.870 \pm 0.031}$	$\mathbf{0.878 \pm 0.027}$

4 Conclusions

In this work, we revisited the well-known patch-based LF framework to propose an improvement that leads to superior performance and considerably reduced runtimes in terms of registration and learning. In most patch-based LF approaches, fusion is carried out in the target space, which requires all training atlases to be spatially transformed to the target image. Extracting patches and their corresponding labels from the atlases' native space instead of using some deformed version after warping them, for instance, to the target space, has shown to be more beneficial. For learning-based approaches, classifiers can be learned offline using the available training atlases and reused in the segmentation of novel target images. Finally, our experiments showed that learning-based LF outperforms similarity-based LF, which reinforces the advantage of using the native patch space due to the added computational advantages that it implies for the learning-based LF.

Acknowledgments. This work is co-financed by the Marie Curie FP7-PEOPLE-2012-COFUND Action, Grant agreement no: 600387.

References

1. Aljabar, P., Heckemann, R., Hammers, A., Hajnal, J., Ruecker, D.: Multi-atlas based segmentation of brain images: atlas selection and its effect on accuracy. NeuroImage **46**(3), 726–738 (2009)
2. Avants, B.B., Epstein, C.L., Grossman, M., Gee, J.C.: Symmetric diffeomorphic image registration with cross-correlation: evaluating automated labeling of elderly and neurodegenerative brain. Med. Image Anal. **12**(1), 26–41 (2008)
3. Bai, W., Shi, W., Ledig, C., Rueckert, D.: Multi-atlas segmentation with augmented features for cardiac MR images. Med. Image Anal. **19**(1), 98–109 (2015)
4. Coupé, P., Manjón, J.V., Fonov, V., Pruessner, J., Robles, M., Collins, D.L.: Patch-based segmentation using expert priors: application to hippocampus and ventricle segmentation. NeuroImage **54**(2), 940–954 (2011)
5. Hao, Y., Wang, T., Zhang, X., Duan, Y., Yu, C., Jiang, T., Fan, Y., for the Alzheimer's Disease Neuroimaging Initiative: Local label learning (LLL) for subcortical structure segmentation: application to hippocampus segmentation. Hum. Brain Mapp. 35(6), 2674–2697 (2014)
6. Rousseau, F., Habas, P.A., Studholme, C.: A supervised patch-based approach for human brain labeling. IEEE Trans. Med. Imaging **30**(10), 1852–1862 (2011)
7. Sanroma, G., Benkarim, O.M., Piella, G., Wu, G., Zhu, X., Shen, D., Ballester, M.Á.G.: Discriminative dimensionality reduction for patch-based label fusion. In: Bhatia, K.K., Lombaert, H. (eds.) MLMMI 2015. LNCS, vol. 9487, pp. 94–103. Springer, Cham (2015). doi:10.1007/978-3-319-27929-9_10
8. Tong, T., Wolz, R., Coup, P., Hajnal, J.V., Rueckert, D.: Segmentation of MR images via discriminative dictionary learning and sparse coding: application to hippocampus labeling. NeuroImage **76**, 11–23 (2013)

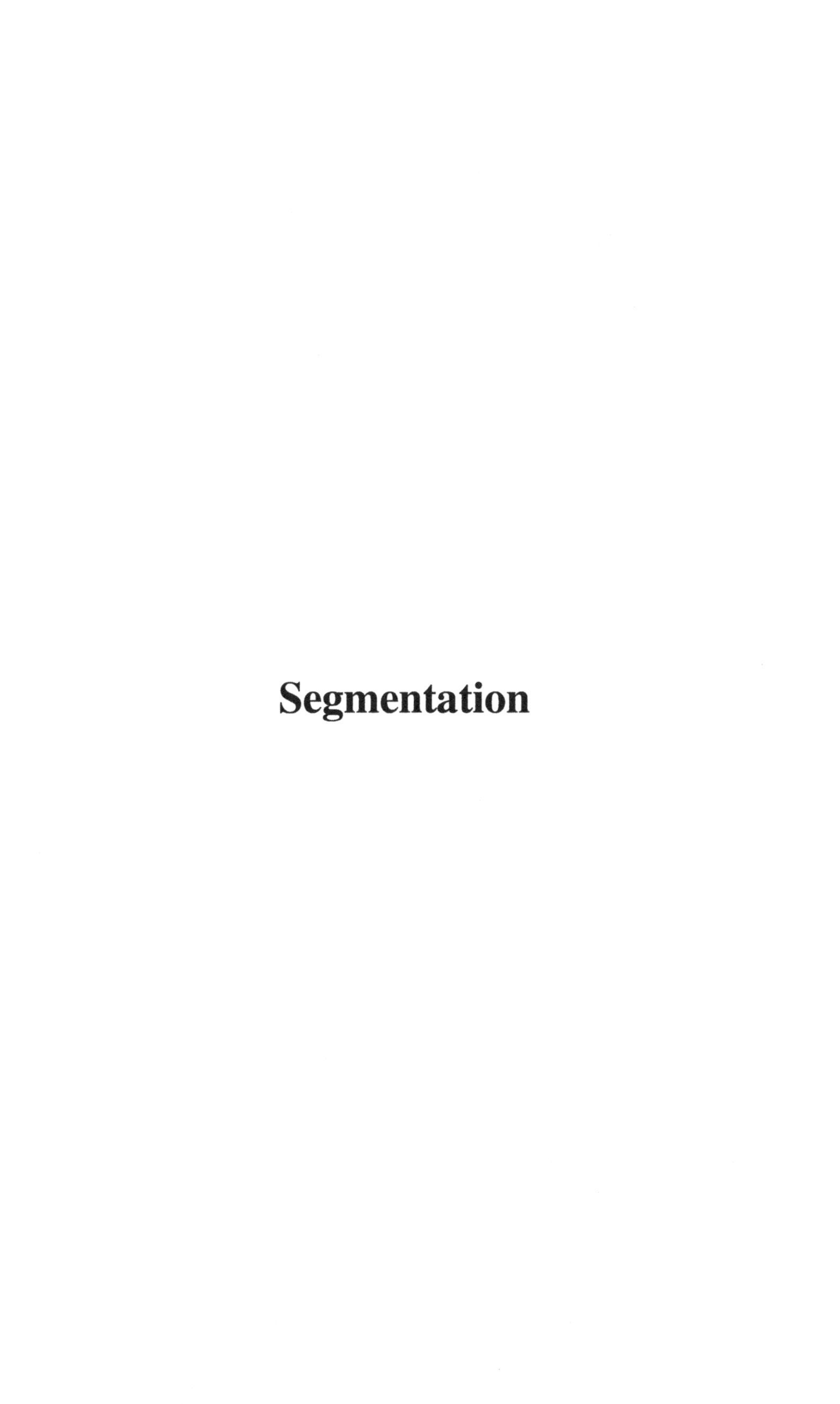

Segmentation

Learning a Sparse Database for Patch-Based Medical Image Segmentation

Moti Freiman[1(✉)], Hannes Nickisch[2], Holger Schmitt[2], Pal Maurovich-Horvat[3], Patrick Donnelly[4], Mani Vembar[5], and Liran Goshen[1]

[1] GAT, CT, Philips Healthcare, Haifa, Israel
moti.freiman@philips.com
[2] Philips Research, Hamburg, Germany
[3] Heart and Vascular Center, Semmelweis University, Budapest, Hungary
[4] South Eastern Health and Social Care Trust, Queen's University, Belfast, Ireland
[5] Clinical Science, CT, Philips Healthcare, Cleveland, OH, USA

Abstract. We introduce a functional for the learning of an optimal database for patch-based image segmentation with application to coronary lumen segmentation from coronary computed tomography angiography (CCTA) data. The proposed functional consists of fidelity, sparseness and robustness to small-variations terms and their associated weights. Existing work address database optimization by prototype selection aiming to optimize the database by either adding or removing prototypes according to a set of predefined rules. In contrast, we formulate the database optimization task as an energy minimization problem that can be solved using standard numerical tools. We apply the proposed database optimization functional to the task of optimizing a database for patch-base coronary lumen segmentation. Our experiments using the publicly available MICCAI 2012 coronary lumen segmentation challenge data show that optimizing the database using the proposed approach reduced database size by 96% while maintaining the same level of lumen segmentation accuracy. Moreover, we show that the optimized database yields an improved specificity of CCTA based fractional flow reserve (0.73 vs 0.7 for all lesions and 0.68 vs 0.65 for obstructive lesions) using a training set of 132 (76 obstructive) coronary lesions with invasively measured FFR as the reference.

Keywords: Energy minimization · Prototype sampling · K-nearest neighbor · Coronary lumen segmentation

1 Introduction

Segmentation of anatomical structures from medical images plays an important role in many clinical applications. Automatic segmentation can be challenging due to the large variability in anatomical structures shape and appearance. Patch-based, non-parametric segmentation algorithms such as the K-nearest neighbor (KNN) algorithm [2] have demonstrated their potential in automatic

© Springer International Publishing AG 2017
G. Wu et al. (Eds.): Patch-MI 2017, LNCS 10530, pp. 47–54, 2017.
DOI: 10.1007/978-3-319-67434-6_6

segmentation of challenging anatomical structures. For example, Mechrez et al. [7] use the KNN algorithm followed by a spatial consistency refinement step to segment Multiple-Sclerosis lesions from MRI data, and Wang et al. [11] demonstrate the potential of KNN algorithm in defining a search-space for improved patch-based segmentation of cardiac MR data and abdominal CT data. Specifically in the cardiovascular domain, Olabarriaga et al. [9] used the KNN algorithm to steer a model-based segmentation of abdominal aortic aneurysms and more recently, Freiman et al. [3] used the KNN algorithm to estimate the likelihood component within a graph min-cut framework for coronary artery lumen segmentation.

While the KNN algorithm has several theoretical and practical advantages [2], two main limitations of this algorithm are: (1) large storage to retain the set of examples which defines the training set, and (2) low efficiency due to the re-calculation of the similarity between the test and training samples at each evaluation [4].

Among the approaches previously proposed to address these issues, database optimization by prototype selection is an attractive approach as it maintains originally an-notated data rather than generating artificial data. The optimal prototype selection is an NP-hard problem which can be mapped onto a set-cover problem and solved using an approximation algorithm [1]. Alternatively, the prototype selection problem can be relaxed by introducing some order on the prototypes. Then, the prototype selection approaches can be divided into three categories: (1) incremental search, in which the algorithm adds prototypes to the reduced data based on some rule, (2) decremental search in which the algorithm aims to remove prototypes from the database according to some rule, and; (3) hybrid approach which combines both incremental and decremental steps. For a comprehensive review of methods aimed to reduce KNN algorithm storage and computational demand we refer the reader to García et al. [4].

In this work we formulate the database optimization problem as an energy minimization which enables the optimization using common numerical approaches. Our functional consists of fidelity, sparsity and robustness to small variations terms along with their associated weights. We applied the proposed functional to optimize a database used in Freiman's et al. patch-based coronary artery lumen segmentation algorithm [3]. We evaluated the influence of database optimization on the segmentation performance by means of segmentation accuracy using the publicly available MICCAI 2012 Coronary Lumen Segmentation Challenge Database [5]. We also evaluated the impact of the database optimization on CCTA based fractional flow reserve (CT-FFR) estimates using a database of 132 coronary lesions with invasively measured FFR as the reference.

Our results show that the database size can be reduced by 96% while maintaining the same level of coronary lumen segmentation accuracy on the MICCAI 2012 Coronary lumen segmentation challenge database [5] and even improving the performance of CT-FFR estimates obtained with 3D models generated from the automatic segmentation results.

2 Method

Our goal is to select a subset of prototypes from a given database so that the classification performance for any new sample will be as accurate as possible. The sub-sampled database should represent the full structure of the population with as few prototypes as possible. First, we define a property describing the distribution of the prototypes in the original database. Next, we define a set of parameters used to generate a sub-sampled database, and finally, we formulate the optimal parameter finding as an energy minimization problem.

2.1 Prototype Ranking

Inspired by the work of Bien and Tibshirani [1], we rank prototypes in the original database according to their location on the manifold. Specifically, we will consider a prototype as located in the center of its class when its neighboring most similar prototypes according to some pre-defined metric are from of the same class and as located on the boundary between classes if it has many neighbors similar samples which are belonging to other from different classes. Formally, for a prototype feature-vector $\boldsymbol{x}$, we define the sample ranking score $R(\boldsymbol{x})$ as follows:

$$R(\boldsymbol{x}) = \frac{\#\text{NN with other class}}{\#\text{NN with same class}} = \frac{\sum_{k=1}^{K} 1 - \delta(C[\boldsymbol{x}], C[\boldsymbol{x_k}])}{\max(\sum_{k=1}^{K} \delta(C[\boldsymbol{x}], C[\boldsymbol{x_k}]), 1)} \tag{1}$$

where K is the number of the nearest prototype neighbors $\boldsymbol{x_i}$ that are similar according to the chosen distance metric, $C[\boldsymbol{x_i}]$ is the class of $\boldsymbol{x_i}$, $\boldsymbol{x}$ is a prototype similar to $\boldsymbol{x_i}$, and:

$$\delta(C[\boldsymbol{x_i}], C[\boldsymbol{x_k}]) = \begin{cases} 1, & C[\boldsymbol{x_i}] = C[\boldsymbol{x_k}] \\ 0, & C[\boldsymbol{x_i}] \neq C[\boldsymbol{x_k}] \end{cases} \tag{2}$$

According to this definition $R(\boldsymbol{x})$ gets a high value when the prototype $\boldsymbol{x}$ has many similar prototypes from other classes, and a low value when the prototype $\boldsymbol{x}$ has many similar prototypes from its own class.

2.2 Database Sparsification

We describe the distribution of the classification sample ranking scores of the prototypes in the original database for each class using a histogram with N bins. The bins boundaries are set (and kept fixed) to be percentiles of the overall samples per class to normalize against various sample ranks distributions. We define a sparsified database as a function of the percentile of prototypes to be selected from each bin of the histogram $DB(\boldsymbol{N})$, where $\boldsymbol{N} \in \mathbb{N}^N$ is the vector containing the number of prototypes to be put in each of the N bins. The subsampling is done deterministically by selecting the N_i prototypes with highest ranking score for bin i.

2.3 Database Optimization

Given the function $DB(\boldsymbol{N})$ to sample the original database, we define a functional to estimate the sampling parameters $\boldsymbol{N}$ i.e. the number of prototypes per bin. Our goal is to find $\boldsymbol{N}$ that maximizes the capability of the sampled database to correctly classify each sample while minimizing the overall number of samples. We also would like the classification to be robust to small variations in the samples. Formally, our functional is defined as:

$$E_{\alpha,\beta}(\boldsymbol{N}) = \sum_{i=1}^{M} \overbrace{\rho(\boldsymbol{N},\boldsymbol{x_i})}^{\text{robustness}} + \alpha \sum_{i=1}^{M} \overbrace{\left(C(\boldsymbol{x_i}) - f\left(DB(\boldsymbol{N}),\boldsymbol{x_i}\right)\right)^2}^{\text{fidelity}} + \beta \overbrace{\|DB(\boldsymbol{N})\|}^{\text{sparsity}} \quad (3)$$

where: $DB(\boldsymbol{N})$ is the sampled database constructed from the original database by sampling the different bins according to the percentiles specified by $\boldsymbol{N}$, $f\left(DB(\boldsymbol{N}),\boldsymbol{x_i}\right)$ is the classification of the prototype $\boldsymbol{x_i}$ using the sampled database $DB(\boldsymbol{N})$, $\|DB(\boldsymbol{N})\|$ is the number of the prototype in the sampled database $DB(\boldsymbol{N})$, M is the number of prototypes in the original database, α,β are weighting meta-parameters controlling the contribution of each term, and $TV(\boldsymbol{N})$ measures the robustness of the the classification of each prototype using $DB(\boldsymbol{N})$ to a small variation in its appearance as follows:

$$\rho(\boldsymbol{N},\boldsymbol{x}) = \sum_{j=1}^{J} \|f\left(DB(\boldsymbol{N}),\boldsymbol{x}\right) - f\left(DB(\boldsymbol{N}),\boldsymbol{x}+\boldsymbol{e_j}\right)\|_1 \quad (4)$$

where J is the dimension of the prototype $\boldsymbol{x}$, the unit vector $\boldsymbol{e_j}$ is of the same dimension as with zeros at all entries except at entry j, and $\|f\left(DB(\boldsymbol{N}),\boldsymbol{x}\right) - f\left(DB(\boldsymbol{N}),\boldsymbol{x}+\boldsymbol{e_j}\right)\|_1$ is the absolute difference between the classification of $\boldsymbol{x}$ and $\boldsymbol{x}+\boldsymbol{e_j}$ given the database $DB(\boldsymbol{N})$.

We find the optimal database sampling parameters by minimizing the energy functional:

$$\hat{\boldsymbol{N}} = \underset{\boldsymbol{N}}{\operatorname{argmin}}\, E_{\alpha,\beta}(\boldsymbol{N}) \quad (5)$$

2.4 Coronary Lumen Segmentation

We apply the proposed approach to reduce the database size required for the coronary lumen segmentation algorithm proposed by Freiman et al. [3]. For the sake of completeness, we briefly describe the relevant parts of the algorithm here. We refer the interested reader to a detailed and complete description provided in [3]. The algorithm formulates the segmentation task as an energy minimization problem over a cylindrical coordinate system [6] where the warped volume along the coronary artery centerline is expressed with the coordinate i representing the index of the cross-sectional plane, and θ, r represent the angle and the radial distance determining a point in the cross-sectional plane

$$E(X) = \sum_{p\in P} \psi_p(x_p) + \lambda \sum_{p,q\in E} \varphi_{p,q}(x_p,x_q) \quad (6)$$

where P is the set of sampled points, x_p is a vertex in the graph representing the point $(i^{x_p}, \theta^{x_p}, r^{x_p})$ sampled from the original CCTA volume, $\psi_p(x_p)$ represents the likelihood of the vertex to belong to the lumen or the background class, p, q are neighboring vertices according to the employed neighboring system E, and $\varphi_{p,q}(x_p, x_q)$ is a penalty for neighboring vertices belonging to different classes ensure the smoothness of the resulted surface. The algorithm uses the KNN algorithm [2] to calculate the likelihood of each vertex x_p belonging to the coronary lumen from a large training database with rays sampled from cardiac CTA data along with manually edited lumen boundary location represented as a binary rays serving as the database prototypes. The likelihood term is additionally adjusted to account for partial volume effects and a $L2$ norm used as the regularization term as described in [3].

2.5 Application of the Database Optimization

The original database used in the coronary lumen segmentation algorithm consists of ~2,130,000 prototypes obtained from 97 CCTA datasets segmented manually by a cardiac CT expert. We consider the lumen radii as the different classes of the rays. We use the L2 norm as the distance metric to define the sample rank (Eq. 1), and experimentally set the number of bins in the histogram N (Eq. 3) to 5. We optimize the functional hyperparameters to achieve the maximal area under the curve (AUC) for CT-FFR estimates with the segmentations obtained using the optimized database with invasive FFR measurements as the reference. Formally, we define a two-phase optimization task, where the outer loop optimized the model hyperparameters α and β:

$$\widehat{\alpha, \beta} = \underset{\alpha,\beta}{\operatorname{argmax}}\, AUC\left(FFR_{CT}\left(DB\left(\boldsymbol{N}\right)\right) - FFR_{GT}\right) \tag{7}$$

and the inner loop find the optimal model parameters for given α, β using Eq. 5. We carried out the optimization using the derivative-free BOBYQA algorithm by Powell [10].

3 Experimental Results

We use two data sets as follows. The first dataset consists of CCTA data of 132 coronary lesions that were retrospectively collected from the medical records of 97 subjects who underwent a CCTA and invasive coronary angiography with invasive FFR measurements due to suspected CAD. CCTA data was acquired using either a Philips Brilliance iCT (gantry rotation time of 0.27 s) or Philips Brilliance 64 (gantry rotation time of 0.42 s). Acquisition mode was either helical retrospective ECG gating (N = 54) or prospectively ECG triggered axial scan (N = 43). The kVp range was 80–140 kVp and the tube output range was 600–1000 mAs for the helical retrospective scans and 200–300 mAs for the prospectively ECG triggered scans.

Cross-sectional area (CSA) based stenosis quantification was performed by an expert reader on 132 lesions, out of which 56 were diagnosed as non-obstructive lesions (CSA stenosis less than 50%) and 76 diagnosed as obstructive lesions (CSA stenosis 50%–90%). According to the invasive FFR measurements, 48 lesions were hemodynamically significant (FFR $\leq$0.8) and 84 lesions were non-significant (FFR $>$ 0.8). The coronary artery centerlines and the aorta segmentation were computed automatically and adjusted manually by a cardiac CT expert (–) to account for algorithm inaccuracies using a commercially available software dedicated to cardiac image analysis (Comprehensive Cardiac Analysis, IntelliSpace Portal 6.0, Philips Healthcare).

We tuned the model hyper-parameters and optimized the database using Eqs. 5 and 7. Next, we segmented the coronary tree with Freiman's et al. algorithm [3] with the full and the optimized databases. Finally, we performed the flow simulations using the lumped parameter model (LM) proposed by Nickisch et al. [8].

We compared the flow simulation results from the 3D coronary tree models generated using the coronary lumen segmentation algorithm described in Sect. 2.4, with the full and optimized training databases. The optimization process reduced the database size by 96% from ~2,130,000 prototypes to ~84,000 prototypes. Figure 1 illustrates the reduction in the number of prototypes in the database at the different bins of the prototypes histogram. The Functional-based optimization prefers to keep prototypes with low sample ratio (i.e. closer to the center of mass of each class) in the optimized database. Table 1 summarizes the performance metrics for assessing the hemodynamic significance of coronary lesions with automatic segmentation using the entire and optimized database for entire set of coronary lesions and specifically for obstructive lesions (Cross Sectional Area (CSA) stenosis $\geq$ 50%). The flow simulation results are slightly

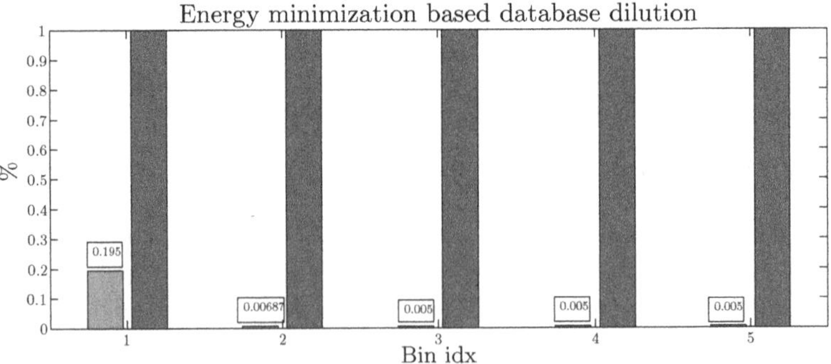

Fig. 1. The database reduction for each bin of the histogram of prototypes. The red bars indicate 100% of the original database and the green bars indicates the percentage of the remaining prototypes after the optimization. Optimized database sampling parameter for each bin is listed above the optimized histogram.(Color figure online)

Table 1. Summary statistics of hemodynamic significance assessment of coronary lesions by means of CT-FRR based on automatic segmentation with the entire database and with the optimized database. Results presented for all (N = 132) lesions and specifically for obstructive (Obst.) lesions (N = 76) separately.

	Sensitivity		Specificity		Accuracy		AUC	
	All	Obst.	All	Obst.	All	Obst.	All	Obst.
Optimized database	0.85	0.86	0.73	0.68	0.77	0.76	0.84	0.83
Full database	0.85	0.86	0.70	0.65	0.76	0.75	0.84	0.82

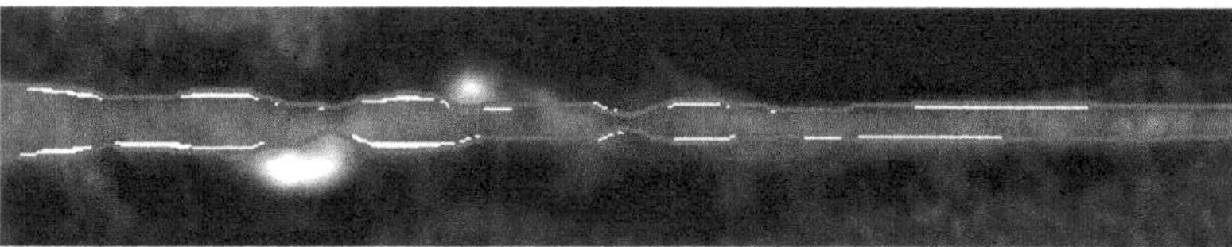

Fig. 2. Representative example of straight multi-planar reconstructed images of coronary artery segmentation results with the optimized (green) and full database.(Color figure online)

Table 2. Summary statistics of coronary lumen segmentation accuracy using the MICCAI 2012 challenge evaluation framework [5] for the training datasets (18 cases, 78 coronary segments). Results presented for healthy and diseased segments separately and in the relevant metric units.

	Dice (%)		MSD (mm)		MAX SD (mm)	
	Healthy	Disease	Healthy	Disease	Healthy	Disease
Optimized database	0.69	0.74	0.49	0.27	1.69	1.24
Full database	0.69	0.74	0.49	0.27	1.69	1.22

better using the optimized database compared to the results of the full database, although the optimized database has much less prototypes compared to the full database.

Figure 2 depicts representative examples of straight multi-planar reconstructed images of coronary artery segmentation results with the optimized (green) and the full (red) database. Table 2 presents the segmentation accuracy results of our algorithm with the original and optimized database using the MICCAI 2012 challenge framework training data [5]. We refer the reader to the challenge website [5] for further comparison with the rest of the methods and with the observer performance.

4 Conclusion

We presented an energy functional for optimizing the training database in patch-based medical image segmentation algorithms. We define a 'sample rank' order on the training database prototypes and formulate the prototype sampling as an energy minimization task with hyper-parameters that can be adjusted to the specific task. We demonstrated the application of this approach to reducing database size and improving the performance of coronary lumen segmentation algorithm from CCTA data. Our experiments show that the optimized database can maintain overall segmentation results with added incremental improvements of CT-FFR estimates based on the 3D models generated from the segmentation results while substantially reducing the memory demand of the algorithm.

References

1. Bien, J., Tibshirani, R.: Prototype selection for interpretable classification. Ann. Appl. Stat. **5**(4), 2403–2424 (2011)
2. Cover, T., Hart, P.: Nearest neighbor pattern classification. IEEE Trans. Inf. Theory **13**(1), 21–27 (1967)
3. Freiman, M., et al.: Improving CCTA-based lesions' hemodynamic significance assessment by accounting for partial volume modeling in automatic coronary lumen segmentation. Med. Phys. **44**(3), 1040–1049 (2017)
4. García, S., et al.: Prototype selection for nearest neighbor classification: taxonomy and empirical study. IEEE Trans. Pattern Anal. Mach. Intell. **34**(3), 417–435 (2012)
5. Kirişli, H., et al.: Standardized evaluation framework for evaluating coronary artery stenosis detection, stenosis quantification and lumen segmentation algorithms in computed tomography angiography. Med. Image Anal. **17**(8), 859–876 (2013). http://coronary.bigr.nl/stenoses/
6. Lugauer, F., Zheng, Y., Hornegger, J., Kelm, B.M.: Precise lumen segmentation in coronary computed tomography angiography. In: Menze, B., Langs, G., Montillo, A., Kelm, M., Müller, H., Zhang, S., Cai, W.T., Metaxas, D. (eds.) MCV 2014. LNCS, vol. 8848, pp. 137–147. Springer, Cham (2014). doi:10.1007/978-3-319-13972-2_13
7. Mechrez, R., Goldberger, J., Greenspan, H.: Patch-based segmentation with spatial consistency: application to MS lesions in brain MRI. Int. J. Biomed. Imaging **2016**, Article ID 7952541 (2016)
8. Nickisch, H., Lamash, Y., Prevrhal, S., Freiman, M., Vembar, M., Goshen, L., Schmitt, H.: Learning patient-specific lumped models for interactive coronary blood flow simulations. In: Navab, N., Hornegger, J., Wells, W.M., Frangi, A. (eds.) MICCAI 2015. LNCS, vol. 9350, pp. 433–441. Springer, Cham (2015). doi:10.1007/978-3-319-24571-3_52
9. Olabarriaga, S.D., et al.: Segmentation of thrombus in abdominal aortic aneurysms from CTA with nonparametric statistical grey level appearance modeling. IEEE Trans. Med. Imaging **24**(4), 477–485 (2005)
10. Powell, M.: The BOBYQA algorithm for bound constrained optimization without derivatives. NA Report NA2009/06, p. 39 (2009). http://www6.cityu.edu.hk/rcms/publications/preprint26.pdf
11. Wang, Z., Bhatia, K.K., Glocker, B., Marvao, A., Dawes, T., Misawa, K., Mori, K., Rueckert, D.: Geodesic patch-based segmentation. In: Golland, P., Hata, N., Barillot, C., Hornegger, J., Howe, R. (eds.) MICCAI 2014. LNCS, vol. 8673, pp. 666–673. Springer, Cham (2014). doi:10.1007/978-3-319-10404-1_83

Accurate and High Throughput Cell Segmentation Method for Mouse Brain Nuclei Using Cascaded Convolutional Neural Network

Qian Wang[1,2(✉)], Shaoyu Wang[2], Xiaofeng Zhu[3], Tianyi Liu[4], Zachary Humphrey[4], Vladimir Ghukasyan[4], Mike Conway[5], Erik Scott[5], Giulia Fragola[4], Kira Bradford[5], Mark J. Zylka[4], Ashok Krishnamurthy[5], Jason L. Stein[4,6], and Guorong Wu[2]

[1] School of Communication and Information Engineering, Xi'an University of Posts and Telecommunications, Xi'an, China
qian_wang@med.unc.edu

[2] BRIC and Department of Radiology, University of North Carolina at Chapel Hill, Chapel Hill, USA

[3] Perelman School of Medicine, University of Pennsylvania, Philadelphia, USA

[4] Neuroscience Center, University of North Carolina, Chapel Hill, USA

[5] Renaissance Computing Institute (RENCI), Chapel Hill, USA

[6] Department of Genetics, University of North Carolina, Chapel Hill, USA

Abstract. Recent innovations in tissue clearing and light sheet microscopy allow rapid acquisition of three-dimensional micron resolution images in fluorescently labeled brain samples. These data allow the observation of every cell in the brain, necessitating an accurate and high-throughput cell segmentation method in order to perform basic operations like counting number of cells within a region; however, large computational challenges given noise in the data and sheer number of features to identify. Inspired by the success of deep learning technique in medical imaging, we propose a supervised learning approach using convolution neural network (CNN) to learn the non-linear relationship between local image appearance (within an image patch) and manual segmentations (cell or background at the center of the underlying patch). In order to improve the segmentation accuracy, we further integrate high-level contextual features with low-level image appearance features. Specifically, we extract contextual features from the probability map of cells (output of current CNN) and train the next CNN based on both patch-wise image appearance and contextual features, extending previous methods into a cascaded approach. Using (a) high-level contextual features extracted from the cell probability map and (b) the spatial information of cell-to-cell locations, our cascaded CNN progressively improves the segmentation accuracy. We have evaluated the segmentation results on mouse brain images, and compared conventional image processing approaches. More accurate and robust segmentation results have been achieved with our cascaded CNN method, indicating the promising potential of our proposed cell segmentation method for use in large tissue cleared images.

© Springer International Publishing AG 2017
G. Wu et al. (Eds.): Patch-MI 2017, LNCS 10530, pp. 55–62, 2017.
DOI: 10.1007/978-3-319-67434-6_7

Keywords: Convolutional neural network · Contextual feature · Cascade learning · Cell segmentation · Mouse microscopy image

1 Introduction

Our understanding of nervous system function is critically dependent on visualizing the three-dimensional structures of the brain. Most critical aspects of cellular identity and functionality, observed at the micron scale and measured by microscopy, are well below the resolution of MRI (Magnetic Resonance Imaging), which acquires images at millimeter resolution. However, higher resolution microscopy images have several computational difficulties such as large image size, low image contrast, and inhomogeneous intensity, which create significant challenges for image analysis.

General speaking, the computational challenges are based on the data size and complexity. A mouse brain (volume of 1000 mm^3) imaged at high resolution (e.g., 0.25 $\mu m \times 0.25\ \mu m \times 1\ \mu m$) results in $\sim$30 TB of data for each fluorescent label [1]. More critically, image quality is usually limited by the image acquisition hardware and scanning time. As shown in Fig. 1, low image contrast (displayed in the red box) and intensity inhomogeneity (displayed in the blue box) are very common which make the conventional image processing methods unable to produce accurate cell segmentation results.

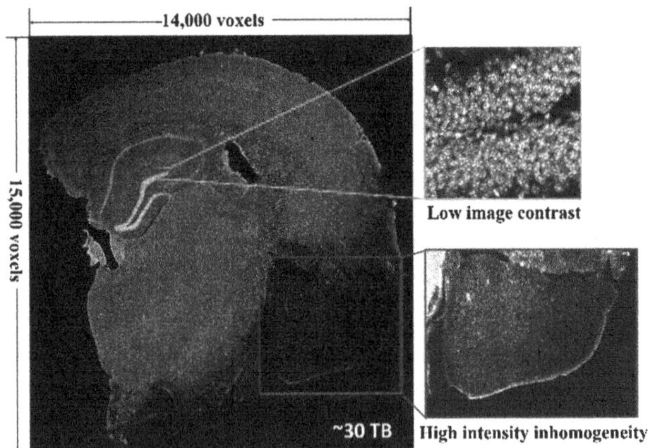

Fig. 1. The challenges in segmenting cells from microscopy image

Current cell detection/segmentation methods are tailored for cell nuclei and use a background subtraction by morphological opening method [1, 2]. Although the computational cost is low for this method, it assumes that the shape of the feature to segment (in this case nuclei) is similar across cell types. This assumption is likely invalid across all cell types (e.g., neuronal nuclei are round whereas endothelial nuclei are oblong) and therefore will result in poor segmentation. Moreover, since each image point in the microcopy image stack is treated equally, such low-level image processing methods are not sufficient to deal with the inhomogeneity issue.

To address above limitations, we propose a novel learning-based segmentation method using convolutional neural networks [3, 4]. Specifically, we first construct a neural network to learn the non-linear mapping between the appearance within the image patch and the label at the center of the underlying image patch, in a layer-by-layer manner. 3D convolution and max pooling techniques [5, 6] are used in training the neural network, which have proven efficient at dealing with high-dimensional volumetric imaging data. In order to address the challenges of poor image contrast and high intensity inhomogeneity, we further proposed to use high-level contextual feature to improve segmentation results. Specifically, the contextual feature representation is extracted from the tentative probability map of cells, which characterize the spatial coordinates with respect to the nearby cells. Then we use both patch-wise image appearance and contextual information to train another CNN, where the input of underlying CNN is the output of previous CNN. With additional high-level contextual features at each voxel, the segmentation can be improved by correcting the possible mis-segmentations by using image appearance features only. Since the contextual features are calculated based on cell probability map produced by the previous CNN, our cascaded CNN can progressively improve the cell segmentation result by refining the contextual features based on the more and more accurate cell probability map. It is worth noting that deep neural network is very suitable for parallel computing such as GPU programming. Hence, our CNN-based cell segmentation method is scalable to apply to microscopy images in current neuroscience studies.

We have evaluated our cascaded CNN in segmenting cells from mouse brain images acquired at the Neuroscience Center at the University of North Carolina at Chapel Hill and imaged on a confocal microscope. Compared with conventional image processing method, our proposed method achieves more accurate and consistent segmentation results in terms of overlap ratio and visual inspection.

2 Methods

To achieve accurate cell segmentation results from a mouse microscopy image, we propose a novel cascaded CNN approach, as shown in Fig. 2. The building block of our proposed segmentation method is a convolutional neural network (the bottom of Fig. 2). In the following, we will first present the CNN based segmentation in Sect. 2.1 and then extend to the cascaded CNN using the contextual feature in Sect. 2.2.

2.1 3D Convolutional Neural Network for Cell Segmentation

Suppose we have a set of image patches $X = \{x_i | i = 1, \ldots, N\}$ and the known label $Y = \{y_i | i = 1, \ldots, N\}$ ($y_i \in \{cell, celledge, background\}$ (manually identified) at the center of image patch. The goal is to learn a non-linear mapping f such that $y_i = f(x_i)$. Since the mapping function f is usually highly complex, we used deep the learning technique to find out the mapping in a layer-by-layer manner, that is, $y_i = f_L(f_{L-1}(\ldots f_1(x_i)))$, where the neural network consists of L layers. Note, there are only

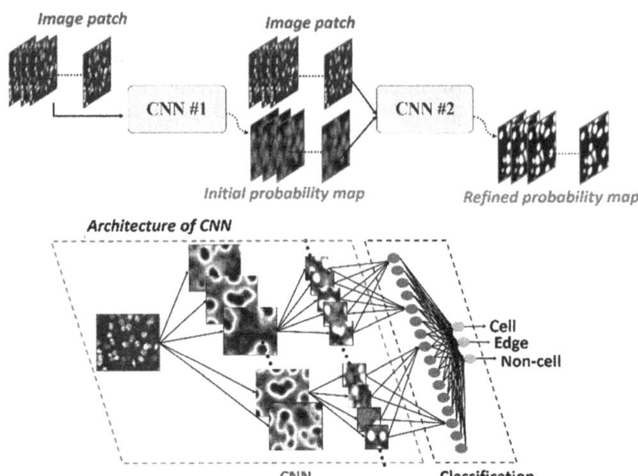

Fig. 2. The overview of our cascaded CNN of cell segmentation method (top) and the architecture of CNN (bottom).

three neurons (green nodes in the bottom of Fig. 2) in the last layer which produce the probability to cell, cell edge, and back ground, respectively. Specifically, Let D and M denote, respectively, the dimensions of hidden representations and input patches. Given an input image patch $x_i \in \mathcal{R}^M$, neural network maps it to be an activation vector $h_i^1 = \left[h_i^1(j)\right]_{j=1,\ldots,D}^T \in \mathcal{R}^D$ by $h_i^1 = f_1(W_1 x_i + b_1)$, where the weight matrix $W_1 \in \mathcal{R}^{D \times L}$ and the bias vector $b_1 \in \mathcal{R}^D$ are the network parameters in the first layer. Here, f is the logistic sigmoid function $f(a) = 1/(1+\exp(-a))$. It is worth noting that h_i^1 is considered as the low-level representation vector of the particular input training patch x_i. Next, the representation h_i^1 from the hidden layer is used as the input of second layer to learn the network parameter W_2 and b_2, where the activation vector h_i^2 encodes the correlations across the low-level features. We repeat the same procedure and construct L layers, as shown in the bottom of Fig. 2. A typical gradient based back-propagation algorithm can be used for fine tuning the network parameters [7, 8].

In order for robustness, the input image patch size is required to be set large enough, e.g., 61 voxels in each dimension. However, it is too complex to learn non-linear mapping in such high dimensional space. Hence, the convolutional technique is employed to reduce the data dimension. The input to the convolutional neural network is the large image patch $\mathcal{P}_v$ with patch size L_v. To make it simple, here, we explain the CNN with a 2D image patch as example. Since the dimension of the image patch $\mathcal{P}_v$ is too large, we let a $L_w \times L_w$ ($L_w < L_v$) sliding window $\mathcal{P}_w$ go through the entire big image patch $\mathcal{P}_v$, thus obtaining $(L_v - L_w + 1) \times (L_v - L_w + 1)$ small image patches. Eventually, we use these small image patches $\mathcal{P}_w$ to train the auto-encoder in each layer, instead of the entire big image patch $\mathcal{P}_v$. Given the parameters of network (weight matrix W_l and bias vector b_l in each layer), we can compute $(L_v - L_w + 1) \times (L_v - L_w + 1)$ activation vectors. Then max pooling [5] is used to shrink the representations by a factor of C in each direction (horizontal or vertical). Specifically, we compute the representative activation vector among these 4 activation vectors in the 2×2 neighborhood by choosing the maximum absolute value for each vector element. Thus, the number of activation vector significantly reduces to $\frac{L_v - L_w + 1}{C} \times \frac{L_v - L_w + 1}{C}$. Since we apply the maximum operation, shrinking the representation with max pooling allows high-level representation to be invariant to small translations of the input image patches and reduce the computational burden.

2.2 Cascaded Convolutional Neural Network Using Contextual Features

In Sect. 2.1, we only use the image appearance information to train CNN. Due to low image contrast, low-level features derived from image intensity are not sufficient to steer the training of neural networks. Other high-level features are of great necessity to alleviate the issue of poor image quality. To this end, we resort to context features [9, 10] which can encode spatial relationship of one structure to other structures.

Since the output of CNN includes the probability of cell at each voxel, we construct patch-wise contextual features based on the tentative cell probability map. It is reasonable to train another CNN using both low-level image appearance and high-level contextual information. Leveraged by the high-level heuristics, we can enhance the reliability of the cell probability map and then use the refined contextual features to train another CNN and so on until the segmentation results converge. Eventually, we turn the conventional CNN method into a cascaded architecture, as shown in the top of Fig. 2. Considering the computation cost, we cascade two CNNs in our experiment.

3 Experiment Results

3.1 Experiment Setting

In the training stage, we randomly sampled $\sim 165{,}000$ training patches to train the cascaded CNN, each image patch with the known label (cell, cell edge, and background) at the patch center. The patch size is set to 61 voxels. Max-pooling of a $2 \times 2 \times 2$ window are operated to combine the activation vectors from convolutional filters.

To evaluate the cell segmentation result, we first compare our cascaded CNN cell segmentation method with classic Otsu's method, where the threshold of intensity is optimized to separate cell and background in the whole image domain. We also apply the enhanced Otsu's method [11], which consider the issue of image artifacts such as noise. Since the main challenge of cell segmentation in microscopy image is from intensity inhomogeneity, we further deploy local Otsu's method where the intensity threshold is adaptive to each local region. Furthermore, we show the cell segmentation results by object detection method [12] using filter convolution technique, which works in the frequency domain and assumes the cell voxels usually have high response to certain specifically designed band-pass filters.

3.2 Results

Advantage of Cascaded CNN Over Single CNN. First, we demonstrate the cell segmentation with and without cascaded architecture. Figure 3(a) and (b) display the original mouse microscopy image and after intensity normalization, where the low illumination in the top-left (red bounding box) makes most of cells in that dark regions being considered as background. The cell probability map by single CNN (use intensity information only) and our cascaded CNN are shown in the Fig. 3(c) and (d), respectively. It is observable that **(1)** learning-based approaches are efficient to alleviate the issue of local intensity inhomogeneity; and **(2)** the cell probability map by cascaded CNN is sharper than single CNN (thus more reliable to binary into cell and background), indicating the advantage of using contextual features and the cascaded architecture.

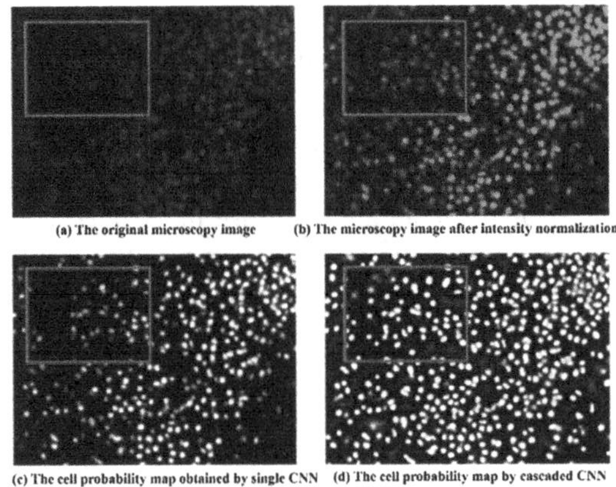

(a) The original microscopy image
(b) The microscopy image after intensity normalization
(c) The cell probability map obtained by single CNN
(d) The cell probability map by cascaded CNN

Fig. 3. The advantage of cascaded CNN over single CNN.

Evaluation of Cell Segmentation Accuracy with Comparison to Current State-of-the-Art Methods. Next, we show the segmentation by classic Otsu's method (using global threshold) in Fig. 4(a), enhanced Otsu's method (using corrected global threshold) in Fig. 4(b), local Otsu's method (using region adaptive threshold) in Fig. 4 (c), band-pass convolution filter in Fig. 4(d), and single CNN (using intensity information only) in Fig. 4(e), and our proposed cascaded CNN (using both intensity and contextual features) in Fig. 4(f), respectively. In general, learning-based approaches outperform the non-learning-based methods via visual inspection. Furthermore, we calculate the overlap degree between the manual segmentation and the automatic cell segmentation result by above six approach. The Dice ratios are shown in Table 1. It is apparent that the improvement by our cascaded CNN is significant in terms of segmentation accuracy.

We test our cell segmentation method on a Dell work station with GPU card (NVIDIA TITAN X with 12 GB frame buffer and 3584 cores @ 1.5 GHz). Without specific program optimization, our cascaded CNN method requires 124 s to complete cell segmentation at a 800×600 image region, voxel by voxel. Future work for speed

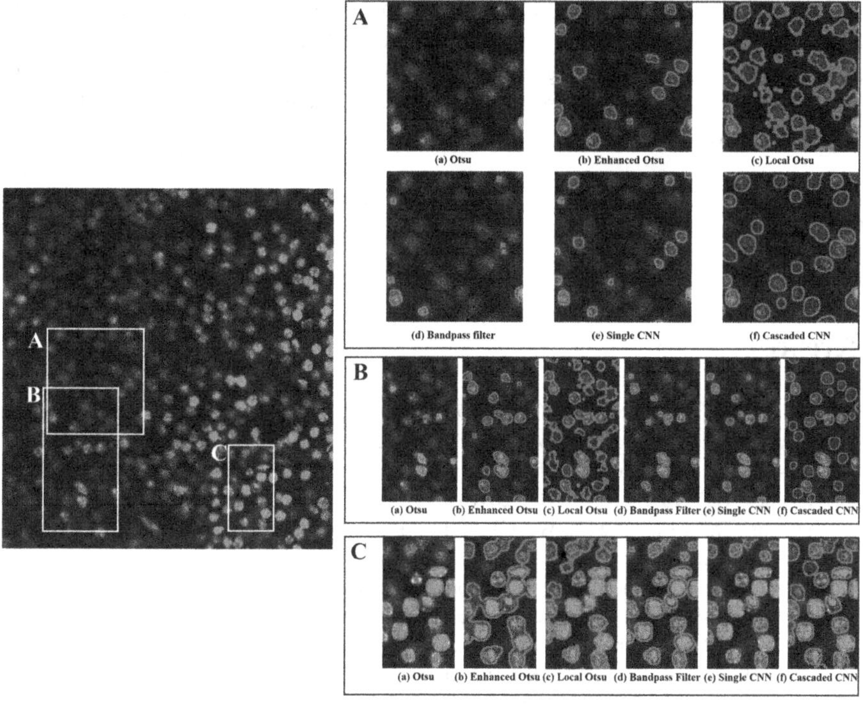

Fig. 4. Cell segmentation result by current state-of-the-art methods and our proposed cascade CNN method.

Table 1. The Dice ratio and computational time by six automatic cell segmentation methods.

Method	Otsu	Enhanced Otsu	Local Otsu	Band-pass filter	Single CNN	Cascaded CNN
Dice	0.421	0.639	0.671	0.576	0.590	0.767
Time(s)	0.303	1.572	3.710	3.756	84.21	124.0

up includes **(1)** fast screening the background points thus we only apply cascaded CNN on difficult-to-segmentation image regions; **(2)** extent current method into multi-resolution framework; **(3)** further optimize the current implementation to fully utilize both CPU and GPU computational resources.

4 Conclusion

In this paper, we propose a novel learning-based nuclear segmentation method for mouse brain microscopy image. Convolutional neural network is used to learn the non-linear mapping between local image appearance and the probability of cell at the center of the underlying patch. In order to address the issues of low image contrast and high intensity inhomogeneity, we further develop the cascaded CNN which utilize both low-level image appearance and high-level contextual features to segment cells out of microscopy image. Promising segmentation results have been achieved which indicates the high potential of our cell segmentation in neuroscience applications like whole brain tissue cleared samples.

Acknowledgements. The research is supported by the National Science Foundation (NSF 1649916). The first author is supported by the China Scholarship Council for one year's visiting at the University of North Carolina at Chapel Hill.

References

1. Renier, N., Adams, E.L., Kirst, C., Wu, Z., Azevedo, R., Kohl, J., Autry, A.E., Kadiri, L., Venkataraju, K.U., Zhou, Y., Wang, V.X., Tang, C.Y., Olsen, O., Dulac, C., Osten, P., Tessier-Lavigne, M.: Mapping of brain activity by automated volume analysis of immediate early genes. Cell **165**, 1789–1802 (2016)
2. Richardson, D.S., Lichtman, J.W.: Clarifying tissue clearing. Cell **162**, 246–257 (2015)
3. Brosch, T., Tang, L.Y.W., Yoo, Y., Li, D.K.B., Traboulsee, A., Tam, R.: Deep 3D convolutional encoder networks with shortcuts for multiscale feature integration applied to multiple sclerosis lesion segmentation. IEEE Trans. Med. Imaging **35**, 1229–1239 (2016)
4. Moeskops, P., Viergever, M.A., Mendrik, A.M., de Vries, L.S., Benders, M.J.N.L., Išgum, I.: Automatic segmentation of MR brain images with a convolutional neural network. IEEE Trans. Med. Imaging **35**, 1252–1262 (2016)
5. Lee, H., Grosse, R., Ranganath, R., Ng, A.Y.: Convolutional deep belief networks for scalable unsupervised learning of hierarchical representations. In: Proceedings of the 26th Annual International Conference on Machine Learning. pp. 609–616. ACM, Montreal, Quebec, Canada (2009)
6. Liu, F., Yang, L.: A novel cell detection method using deep convolutional neural network and maximum-weight independent set. In: Navab, N., Hornegger, J., Wells, William M., Frangi, Alejandro F. (eds.) MICCAI 2015. LNCS, vol. 9351, pp. 349–357. Springer, Cham (2015). doi:10.1007/978-3-319-24574-4_42
7. Arnold, L., Rebecchi, S., Chevallier, S., Paugam-moisy, H.: An introduction to deep-learning. In: European Symposium on Artificial Neural Networks in Computational Intelligence and Machine Learning (ESANN) (2011)
8. Bengio, Y., Courville, A., Vincent, P.: Representation learning: a review and new perspectives. Arxiv arXiv:1206.5538 (2012)
9. Kim, M., Wu, G., Guo, Y., Shen, D.: Joint labeling of multiple Regions of Interest (ROIs) by enhanced auto context models. In: 2015 IEEE International Symposium on Biomedical Imaging (ISBI), New York (2015)
10. Tu, Z., Bai, X.: Auto-context and its application to high-level vision tasks and 3D brain image segmentation. IEEE Trans. Pattern Anal. Mach. Intell. **21**, 1744–1757 (2010)
11. Sezgin, M., Sankur, B.: Survey over image thresholding techniques and quantitative performance evaluation. J. Electron. Imaging **13**, 146–165 (2004)
12. Ghamisi, P., Couceiro, M.S., Martins, F.M.L., Benediktsson, J.A.: Multilevel image segmentation based on fractional-order darwinian particle swarm optimization. IEEE Trans. Geosci. Remote Sens. **52**, 2382–2395 (2014)

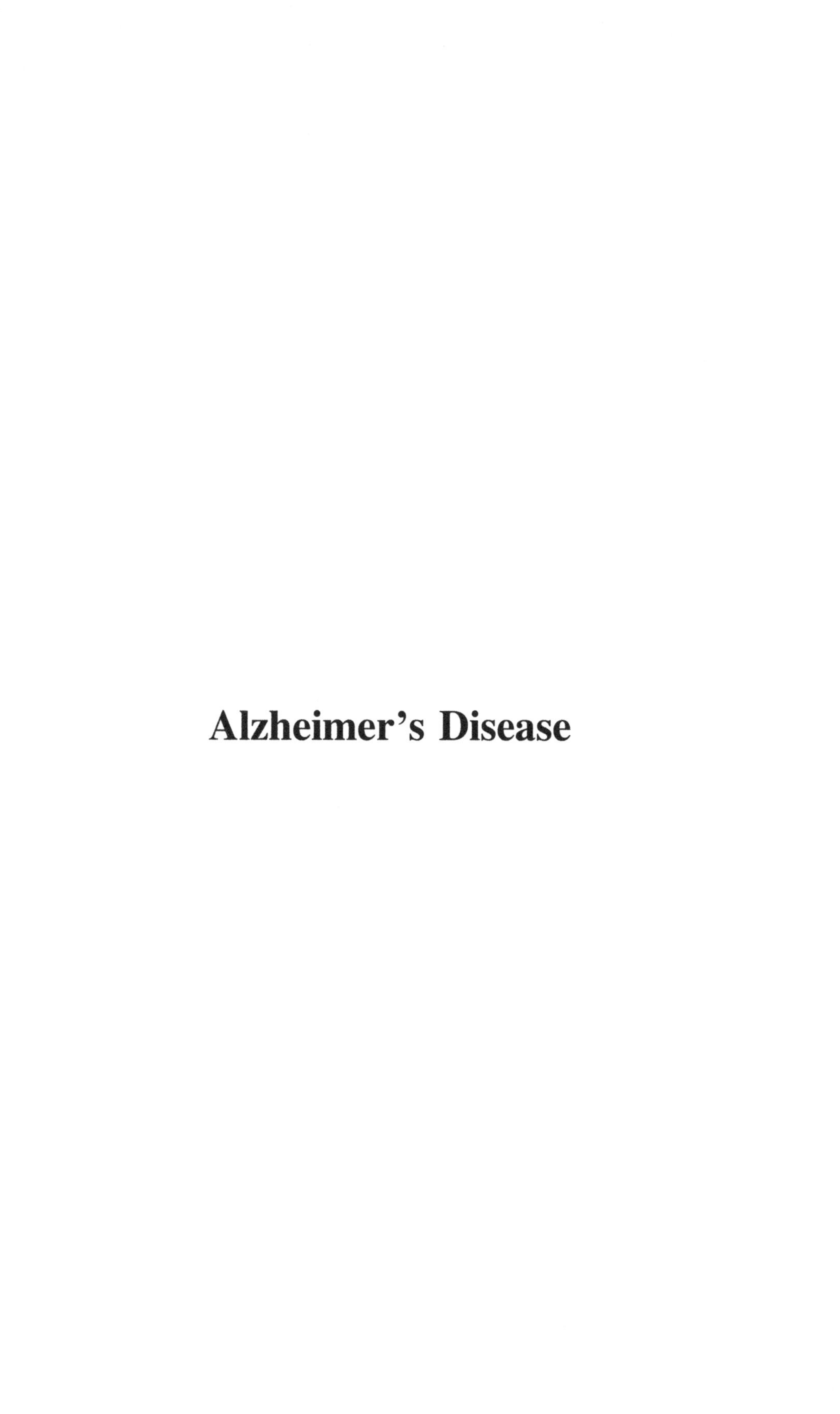

Alzheimer's Disease

Learning-Based Estimation of Functional Correlation Tensors in White Matter for Early Diagnosis of Mild Cognitive Impairment

Lichi Zhang[1], Han Zhang[1], Xiaobo Chen[1], Qian Wang[2], Pew-Thian Yap[1], and Dinggang Shen[1(✉)]

[1] Department of Radiology and BRIC, University of North Carolina at Chapel Hill, Chapel Hill, NC, USA
dgshen@med.unc.edu
[2] Med-X Research Institute, School of Biomedical Engineering, Shanghai Jiao Tong University, Shanghai, China

Abstract. It has been recently demonstrated that the local BOLD signals in resting-state fMRI (rs-fMRI) can be captured for the white matter (WM) by functional correlation tensors (FCTs). FCTs provide similar orientation information as diffusion tensors (DTs), and also functional information concerning brain dynamics. However, FCTs are susceptible to noise due to the low signal-to-noise ratio nature of WM BOLD signals. Here we introduce a robust FCT estimation method to facilitate individualized diagnosis. *First*, we develop a noise-tolerating patch-based approach to measure spatiotemporal correlations of local BOLD signals. *Second*, it is also enhanced by DTs predicted from the input rs-fMRI using a learning-based regression model. We evaluate our trained regressor using the high-resolution HCP dataset. The regressor is then applied to estimate the robust FCTs for subjects in the ADNI2 dataset. We demonstrate for the first time the disease diagnostic value of robust FCTs.

1 Introduction

Resting-state functional magnetic resonance imaging (rs-fMRI) has been widely applied as the non-invasive imaging technique for studying the human brain functional organization architecture. It was originally designed to detect the variations and covariations of the blood-oxygenation-level-dependent (BOLD) signals mostly related to the spontaneous neural activities [1]. The majority of rs-fMRI studies focus on the gray matter (GM), while the rs-fMRI signals in white matter (WM) pathways are treated as noise and artifacts. However, recent studies indicate that WM may also contain meaningful BOLD signals, which carry potentially valuable information complementary to GM-based rs-fMRI studies. Nevertheless, utilizing WM BOLD signals for basic and clinical neuroscience studies is challenging, as WM has blood vasculature that is much less denser, and also the BOLD signal in WM is significantly weaker than in GM [2].

Despite the challenges, attempts have been made to investigate WM fMRI. Early task-based fMRI studies have revealed consistent, reliable task activations in several corpus callosal WM areas linking activated GM structures [3, 4]. Recently, Ding *et al.*

© Springer International Publishing AG 2017
G. Wu et al. (Eds.): Patch-MI 2017, LNCS 10530, pp. 65–73, 2017.
DOI: 10.1007/978-3-319-67434-6_8

[5] found WM functional anisotropic patterns using local functional connectivity (FC) using rs-fMRI, which grossly resemble the anisotropic diffusivity reflected by diffusion tensor imaging (DTI) in several major WM structures. They employed functional correlation tensor (FCT) to capture such anisotropy, allowing functional WM tractography based on rs-fMRI data of a small group of healthy subjects. However, it is challenging when applied to other large cohorts, owing to the limited signal-to-noise ratio (SNR) of the WM BOLD signals. Moreover, the FCT estimation method proposed in [5] does not leverage any prior knowledge of DT data that can help overcome the SNR issue. Thus, a robust and reliable FCT estimation technique is important for greater utility of WM anisotropy in neuroscience studies and also as biomarkers for disease diagnosis.

In this paper, we propose a robust FCT estimation technique to address the aforementioned issues. *First*, we develop a novel patch-based correlation measurement strategy to suppress noise. *Second*, we propose to leverage the underlying WM fiber orientation information as prior knowledge when calculating the FCT. This is based on the finding that the dominant direction of the local WM FC anisotropic pattern, extracted from rs-fMRI, is roughly consistent with that of the diffusion tensors (DTs) from DTI [5] in major WM fiber structures. Thus, we can improve FCT estimation by increasing weighting along the dominant directions of DTs. Ideally, the DTs can be obtained from DTI [6]. In the case where DTI is not available, we employ a learning based method to predict the DTs from the rs-fMRI data. This is achieved by using random forest regression with cascaded learning strategy [7] to learn the FC-to-DT mapping [8, 9] with a training dataset containing both rs-fMRI and DTI. Thus, for a testing rs-fMRI, the learned mapping can be applied to predict DTs. Also note that to consider between-tissue difference, the tissue probability features of GM/WM/cerebrospinal fluid (CSF) from T1-weighted MRI are also used to guide the FC-to-DT mapping process.

2 Materials and Methods

Two datasets are employed in this paper: (1) The Human Connectome Project (HCP) [10] dataset and (2) the Alzheimer's Disease Neuroimaging Initiative Phase-II (ADNI2) dataset [11]. The HCP dataset contains high spatial and temporal resolution rs-fMRI, multi-shell diffusion MRI data, and T1-weighted MRI for each subject. It is hence suitable for training the regression model. The ADNI2 dataset focuses on capturing the progression of mild cognitive impairment (MCI) and early Alzheimer's disease (AD) with both rs-fMRI and T1 MRI. It contains data for early MCI patients, which are used for validation of the improved FCTs in enhancing AD diagnosis.

2.1 Data Preprocessing

HCP Dataset: We randomly select 96 subjects from the dataset, which are all scanned with a customized Siemens Skyra 3T scanner with the same imaging parameters (rs-fMRI: voxel size = $2 \times 2 \times 2$ mm^3, 1200 volumes; DTI: voxel size = $1.25 \times 1.25 \times 1.25$ mm^3; T1: $0.7 \times 0.7 \times 0.7$ mm^3). Note that the first 30 frames in the rs-fMRI images are discarded for magnetization equilibrium. The first 600 frames (7 min and 12 s) of the remaining data are used to estimate FCTs. The preprocessing of the rs-fMRI and DTI data is based on the HCP pipeline (https://github.com/Washington-University/Pipelines), but modified for our requirements as below:

(1) The DTs are computed using *dtifit* in FSL [12]. An average *b*0 image is used for inter-modality registration to rs-fMRI using *flirt* in FSL.
(2) The tissue probability maps for GM/WM/CSF segmentation are obtained from the T1 MRI by using *fast* in FSL, and are linearly warped to each subject's own rs-fMRI space using *flirt*.
(3) FCT computation is performed in the native space of the rs-fMRI per subject. The DTs are warped to each subject's own rs-fMRI space.
(4) The minimally preprocessed rs-fMRI (in native space) are further band-pass filtered ($0.01 \leq f \leq 0.08$ Hz). No spatial smoothing is applied. All subjects' head motion profiles are checked to ensure that they are within an acceptable range.

ADNI2 Dataset: 39 early-stage MCI (eMCI) and 42 age- and gender-matched normal controls (NC) are included. The rs-fMRI (TR = 3000 ms, 140 frames, voxel size = $3.3 \times 3.3 \times 3.3$ mm^3, eyes open) and T1 MRI (voxel size = $1 \times 1 \times 1$ mm^3) are obtained using 3T Phillips Achieva scanners. Data preprocessing is conducted based on SPM8 (https://www.fil.ion.ucl.ac.uk/spm/soft-ware/spm8/), REST (http://www.restfmri.net/forum/REST_V1.8), and DPARSFA (http://rfmri.org/DPARSF) tool boxes with similar procedures as those used for HCP data. T1 MRI is also segmented and coregistered to each subject's native rs-fMRI space. No subject's head motion exceeds 2 mm or 2°.

2.2 Regression Forest for FC-to-DT Mapping

We describe here how the DT-like tensors can be estimated from the HCP rs-fMRI data, and how the learned DT-like tensors can be used to guide FCT estimation using the ADNI2 rs-fMRI data. In the training stage, we extract features from randomly selected 3D patches. Using the obtained patch feature vectors, the regression forest method is trained to predict the corresponding DT at a center voxel of each patch. In the testing stage, the trained regression model is applied patch-wise to the input image to estimate DT-like tensors.

The feature vector is composed of two types of features: (1) local FC from rs-fMRI and (2) tissue probability maps of WM/GM/CSF from T1 MRI. For rs-fMRI, we follow [5] for computing the local FC as the *correlation features*. Specifically, we compute the Pearson's correlation coefficients between the center voxel and its neighboring voxels. Note that, unlike [5], we also include voxels beyond the neighboring 26 voxels. For each of the three probability maps obtained from T1 MRI, we use the 3D Haar-like operators [9] to compute *tissue-probability features*. These two types of the features extracted from the two modalities are then concatenated as a single feature vector.

The process of training the regression forest generally follows the steps in [8, 9]. The major difference here is in the splitting function that is used to split the patch samples in the current node into the left and right child nodes. The criterion of the splitting function is based on one feature selected by exhaustive search within the feature subset, which can maximize the information gain of the splitted groups of training patches based on their corresponding target values. Specifically, the target DT information can be formatted as a 3×3 symmetric matrix, which includes six effective components and can be reshaped as a DT vector; therefore, the splitting function produces six estimates of the information gain corresponding to the six elements of the DT target, which are then averaged as an overall information gain to guide the splitting. In this way, the forest method can gauge all the information in the target vector for training the regressor. It is worth noting that, by combining tissue probability-based features, DT-like tensors can be estimated with more accuracy, because the local FC patterns in the GM and WM could be different, and accordingly the "FC-to-DT" mapping for GM voxels could also be different from the "FC-to-DT" mapping for WM voxels. Our experiment has shown that, by adding tissue-specific features, the testing rs-fMRI data can generate much better DT-like tensor maps.

It is worth noting that we also incorporate the auto-context model [7, 9] as cascade learning strategy for helping improving the mapping performance. Specifically, we refine the mapping by cascading multiple stages of regressions. The first-stage regressor uses only the correlation and tissue-probability features, while, in the subsequent stages, the *context* features obtained from the DTs predicted in the previous stage are also considered. Since each DT consist of six elements, the *context* features are computed using Haar-like operators for each DT element and then concatenated together.

2.3 FCT Estimation

We use the ADNI2 data to calculate the FCT with the guidance from the DTs predicted from the rs-fMRI data with the learned mapping model (using the HCP rs-fMRI data). For each voxel V_i from the input rs-fMRI data, the FCT $\boldsymbol{T}_i$ is represented using a 3×3 symmetric matrix, which is in the same mathematical form as the DT:

$$\boldsymbol{T}_i = \begin{bmatrix} T_{xx} & T_{xy} & T_{xz} \\ T_{xy} & T_{yy} & T_{yz} \\ T_{xz} & T_{yz} & T_{zz} \end{bmatrix}. \tag{1}$$

To estimate it, the first step is to compute the Pearson's correlation coefficient C_{ij} between the center voxel V_i and each of its 26 neighboring voxels V_j. To increase the robustness of such a process to the noise and artifacts in rs-fMRI, we follow a patch-based strategy to implement the correlation measurement. Denote Q_i and Q_j as the two $k \times k \times k$ patches centered at voxel V_i and V_j, respectively. Here, we set $k = 3$ which suits the spatial resolution of the mostly-adopted rs-fMRI data such as in the ADNI dataset. The correlation coefficient C_{ij} is therefore given as

$$C_{ij} = \frac{\sum_{x=1}^{k}\sum_{y=1}^{k}\sum_{z=1}^{k} b(x,y,z) f_{\text{corr}}\left(Q_i(x,y,z), Q_j(x,y,z)\right)}{\sum_{x=1}^{k}\sum_{y=1}^{k}\sum_{z=1}^{k} b(x,y,z)}, \tag{2}$$

where $Q(x,y,z)$ is the voxel at location (x,y,z) of the patch Q, $f_{\text{corr}}(V_i, V_j)$ is the Pearson's correlation comparing the time courses of V_i and V_j, $b(x,y,z) = \exp\left(-\frac{(x-\mu)^2+(y-\mu)^2+(z-\mu)^2}{2\rho^2}\right)$ is the Gaussian kernel used for weighting the correlations, with $\mu = (k+1)/2$ and ρ as a scaling coefficient. In our study, $\rho^2 = 1.25$ gives the optimal results.

Next, we compute a unit vector $\mathbf{n}_{ij} = \{n_{ij,1}, n_{ij,2}, n_{ij,3}\}$ describing the direction from the center voxel V_i to each of its neighbors V_j, the dyadic tensor $\boldsymbol{D}_{ij}$ is given as

$$\boldsymbol{D}_{ij} = \begin{pmatrix} n_{ij,1}\cdot n_{ij,1} & n_{ij,1}\cdot n_{ij,2} & n_{ij,1}\cdot n_{ij,3} \\ n_{ij,2}\cdot n_{ij,1} & n_{ij,2}\cdot n_{ij,2} & n_{ij,2}\cdot n_{ij,3} \\ n_{ij,3}\cdot n_{ij,1} & n_{ij,3}\cdot n_{ij,2} & n_{ij,3}\cdot n_{ij,3} \end{pmatrix}. \tag{3}$$

Third, the orientation information derived from the DT-like tensors is calculated by applying an orientation distribution function (ODF) [13] to obtain the weighting function $\beta(\mathbf{n}_{ij}) = 1/\left(4\pi Z|\boldsymbol{B}|^{\frac{1}{2}}\left(\mathbf{n}_{ij}^{\mathrm{T}}\boldsymbol{B}^{-1}\mathbf{n}_{ij}\right)^{\frac{3}{2}}\right)$, where Z is a normalization constant and $\boldsymbol{B}$ is the learned DT represented using a 3×3 symmetric matrix.

Finally, we compute the robust FCT $\boldsymbol{T}_i$ by summing up all the dyadic tensors $\boldsymbol{D}_{ij}$ with their respective correlation coefficients C_{ij} and corresponding weighting coefficients $\beta(\mathbf{n}_{ij})$:

$$\boldsymbol{T}_i = \sum\nolimits_j C_{ij}\boldsymbol{D}_{ij}\,\beta(\mathbf{n}_{ij}). \tag{4}$$

In this way, the dyadic tensors along with the main directions of DT-like tensor have higher weights in $\beta(\mathbf{n}_{ij})$ than those at other directions. The overall framework of FCT computation is summarized in Fig. 1.

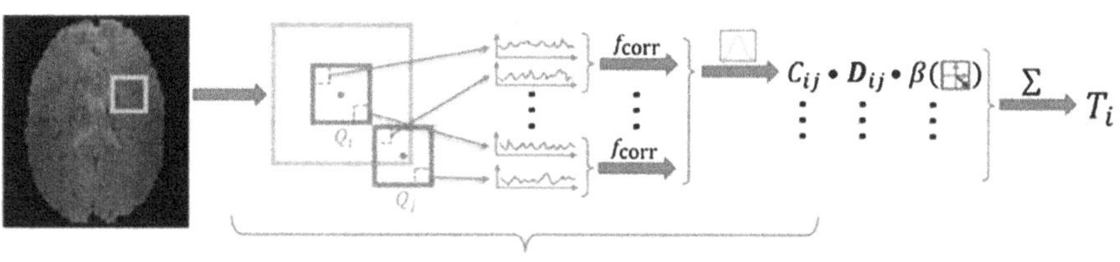

Fig. 1. The overall pipeline for robust FCT computation.

3 Experimental Results

We demonstrate the validity of our proposed framework by evaluating both the learned DT-like tensors and the final FCTs. For the HCP dataset that is used to learn the regression model, we first show the accuracy of the learned DT-like tensors by comparing them with the actual DTs derived from DTI. This is done using 4-fold cross-validation on the HCP dataset. The parameters for training the regression model are identical in all folds. From each rs-fMRI data, we extract 20000 patches with the size of $11 \times 11 \times 11$ in voxels. The number of correlation features for each patch is set to be 1000, and the number of tissue-probability features for each segmented ROI is also set to be 1000. The trained regression forest has 20 trees, and the minimum sample number for the leaf node is set as 8. Note that when implementing the cascaded learning strategy, we connect three regression models. The maximum of the tree depth is 30 in the first regression model as it is trained without context features, and 33 for each of the later stages.

We evaluate the similarity between the predicted DTs in different stages of the cascade and the actual DTs by measuring Pearson's correlations of their fractional anisotropy (FA) maps. The overall correlation coefficients without the cascade is 0.877 $\pm$ 0.015, which is improved to 0.894 $\pm$ 0.015 with the cascade. This shows the validity of the mapping and the effectiveness of the cascade. Furthermore, Fig. 2 shows the FA maps computed from the predicted DTs using the two different configurations, as well as the actual FA map from DTI for reference.

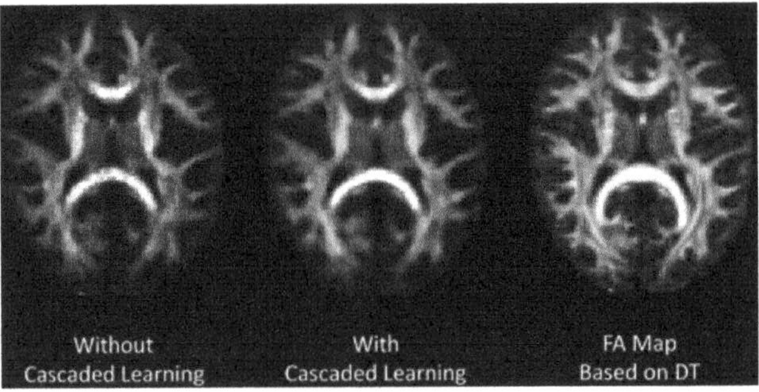

Fig. 2. The FA maps from the DTI-like tensors and actual DTI (used as reference).

In the second experiment, we show the generalizability of the trained regression model (based on the HCP dataset), by directly applying it to the ADNI2 dataset for robust FCT estimation. Figure 3 shows the FA maps using the original FCT calculation method proposed in [5] and using our proposed FCT estimation method. It can be observed that noise is significantly reduced with our method, and the estimated FA map is more reasonable, i.e., with high FA values in the major WM structures (such as the genu and splenium parts of corpus callosum) compared with the FA in the GM regions.

In the third experiment, we further evaluate the validity of our method by applying the resultant FCTs from both eMCI and NC subjects in ADNI2 as features for early AD

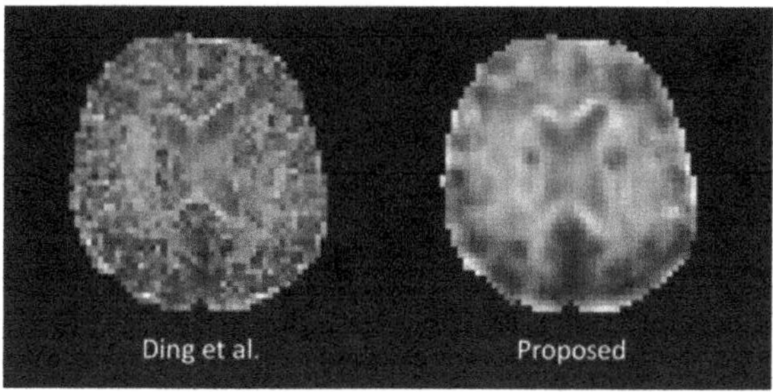

Fig. 3. The FA maps of the obtained FCTs using the method of Ding et al. (left) and our proposed method (right).

diagnosis. Specifically, given the FA maps computed in the native space from the FCTs based on rs-fMRI of ADNI2, SPM8 is used to non-rigidly register them to the standard MNI-152 space. Next, an in-house WM fiber bundle probability template, consisting of 359 major WM segments linking 359 pairs of Automated Anatomical Labeling (AAL) brain regions and generated based on the DTI data of 500 subjects in HCP, is applied to each subject's registered FA map. The fiber-probability-weighted average FA and the weighted variance of FA values in each of the 359 WM segments are computed as features for subsequent classification. In this way, each subject has two 359-by-1 feature vectors (corresponding to the weighted mean FA and the weighted FA variance obtained from FCTs). LASSO-based feature selection [14] is conducted to the two feature vectors separately. Two support vector machine (SVM) classifiers [15] are then trained, respectively. The prediction scores from the two classifiers are fused to give a final classification result. Leave-one-out cross-validation is used to evaluate classification performance.

Experiments show that using FCTs from rs-fMRI, even extracted from only several major WM structures and fed into a simple classifier, the accuracy (ACC) and the area-under-curve (AUC) for eMCI classification still reach the satisfactory level (i.e.,

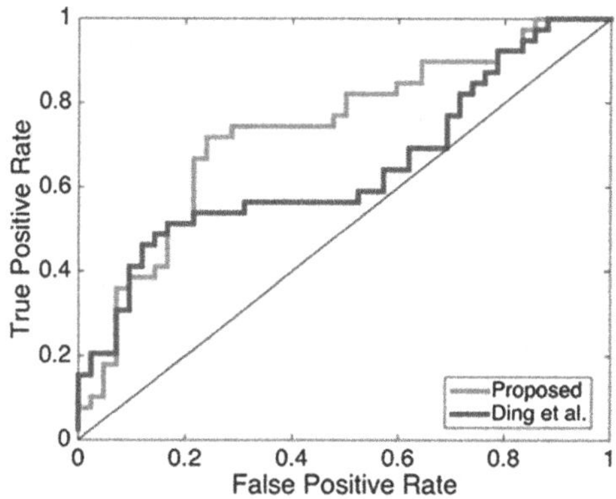

Fig. 4. The ROC curve for the eMCI-NC classification using Ding et al.'s method and our proposed method, respectively.

72.84% and 73.63%, respectively). On the other hand, if using the original FCT calculation method [5], the performance is relatively low (i.e., ACC = 67.90% and AUC = 64.53%). The improvements by our proposed FCT calculation method are also visualized using ROC curves in Fig. 4.

4 Conclusion

In this work, we have presented a novel framework for robust FCT estimation. First, based on high-resolution rs-fMRI and DTI data, we employ regression forest for predicting DTs by using *both* local temporal correlation features from rs-fMRI *and* tissue-probability features from T1 MRI. Then, the predicted DTs are further used as a prior to improve FCT estimation. In the experiments, we have also demonstrated that the resulting FCTs can be used as features for diagnosis of eMCI.

References

1. Gore, J.C.: Principles and practice of functional MRI of the human brain. J. Clin. Investig. **112**, 4–9 (2003)
2. Wise, R.G., Ide, K., Poulin, M.J., Tracey, I.: Resting fluctuations in arterial carbon dioxide induce significant low frequency variations in BOLD signal. Neuroimage **21**, 1652–1664 (2004)
3. Tettamanti, M., Paulesu, E., Scifo, P., Maravita, A., Fazio, F., Perani, D., Marzi, C.: Interhemispheric transmission of visuomotor information in humans: fMRI evidence. J. Neurophysiol. **88**, 1051–1058 (2002)
4. Mosier, K.M., Liu, W.-C., Maldjian, J.A., Shah, R., Modi, B.: Lateralization of cortical function in swallowing: a functional MR imaging study. Am. J. Neuroradiol. **20**, 1520–1526 (1999)
5. Ding, Z., Xu, R., Bailey, S.K., Wu, T.-L., Morgan, V.L., Cutting, L.E., Anderson, A.W., Gore, J.C.: Visualizing functional pathways in the human brain using correlation tensors and magnetic resonance imaging. Magn. Reson. Imaging **34**, 8–17 (2016)
6. Basser, P.J., Pajevic, S., Pierpaoli, C., Duda, J., Aldroubi, A.: In vivo fiber tractography using DT-MRI data. Magn. Reson. Med. **44**, 625–632 (2000)
7. Tu, Z., Bai, X.: Auto-context and its application to high-level vision tasks and 3D brain image segmentation. IEEE Trans. Pattern Anal. Mach. Intell. **32**, 1744–1757 (2010)
8. Criminisi, A., Shotton, J., Konukoglu, E.: Decision forests: a unified framework for classification, regression, density estimation, manifold learning and semi-supervised learning. Found Trends® Comput. Graph. Vis. **7**, 81–227 (2012)
9. Zhang, L., Wang, Q., Gao, Y., Wu, G., Shen, D.: Automatic labeling of MR brain images by hierarchical learning of atlas forests. Med. Phys. **43**, 1175–1186 (2016)
10. Van Essen, D.C., Smith, S.M., Barch, D.M., Behrens, T.E.J., Yacoub, E., Ugurbil, K., Consortium, W.U.-M.H.: The WU-Minn human connectome project: an overview. Neuroimage **80**, 62–79 (2013)
11. Mueller, S.G., Weiner, M.W., Thal, L.J., Petersen, R.C., Jack, C., Jagust, W., Trojanowski, J.Q., Toga, A.W., Beckett, L.: The Alzheimer's disease neuroimaging initiative. Neuroimaging Clin. N. Am. **15**, 869–877 (2005)

12. Jenkinson, M., Beckmann, C.F., Behrens, T.E., Woolrich, M.W., Smith, S.M.: FSL. Neuroimage **62**, 782–790 (2012)
13. Aganj, I., Lenglet, C., Sapiro, G., Yacoub, E., Ugurbil, K., Harel, N.: Reconstruction of the orientation distribution function in single-and multiple-shell q-ball imaging within constant solid angle. Magn. Reson. Med. **64**, 554–566 (2010)
14. Saeys, Y., Inza, I., Larrañaga, P.: A review of feature selection techniques in bioinformatics. Bioinform. **23**, 2507–2517 (2007)
15. Cortes, C., Vapnik, V.: Support-vector networks. Mach. Learn. **20**, 273–297 (1995)

Early Prediction of Alzheimer's Disease with Non-local Patch-Based Longitudinal Descriptors

Gerard Sanroma[1(✉)], Víctor Andrea[1], Oualid M. Benkarim[1], José V. Manjón[2], Pierrick Coupé[3,4], Oscar Camara[1], Gemma Piella[1], and Miguel A. González Ballester[1,5]

[1] DTIC, Universitat Pompeu Fabra, Barcelona, Spain
gerard.sanroma@upf.edu
[2] ITACA, Universitat Politécnica de Valéncia, Valencia, Spain
[3] University of Bordeaux, LaBRI, UMR 5800, 33400 Talence, France
[4] CNRS, LaBRI, UMR 5800, 33400 Talence, France
[5] ICREA, Pg. Lluis Companys 23, 08010 Barcelona, Spain

Abstract. Alzheimer's disease (AD) is characterized by a progressive decline in the cognitive functions accompanied by an atrophic process which can already be observed in the early stages using magnetic resonance images (MRI). Individualized prediction of future progression to AD, when patients are still in the mild cognitive impairment (MCI) stage, has potential impact for preventive treatment. Atrophy patterns extracted from longitudinal MRI sequences provide valuable information to identify MCI patients at higher risk of developing AD in the future. We present a novel descriptor that uses the similarity between local image patches to encode local displacements due to atrophy between a pair of longitudinal MRI scans. Using a conventional logistic regression classifier, our descriptor achieves 76% accuracy in predicting which MCI patients will progress to AD up to 3 years before conversion.

Keywords: Early AD prediction · Non-local patch-based label fusion · Longitudinal analysis

1 Introduction

Alzheimer's disease (AD) is characterized by a progressive decline of the cognitive abilities. Before being diagnosed as probable AD, patients usually go through a mild cognitive impairment (MCI) stage. The earliest signs of neurodegeneration can be observed using magnetic resonance images (MRI) already at the MCI stage [7]. Machine learning techniques have taken advantage of this fact to characterize individuals at different stages of the disease. Cuingnet *et al.* [6] presented a comparison of 10 methods for discrimination of healthy controls (HC) and AD patients with different degrees of neurodegeneration. The most common MRI-based features used for discrimination include tissue probability maps, cortical thickness, hippocampal morphometry or a combination of them [14].

© Springer International Publishing AG 2017
G. Wu et al. (Eds.): Patch-MI 2017, LNCS 10530, pp. 74–81, 2017.
DOI: 10.1007/978-3-319-67434-6_9

Among the personalized medicine approaches related to AD, the discrimination between patients that will remain stable in the MCI stage (i.e., s-MCI) and the ones that will progress to AD in the future (i.e., p-MCI) is possibly the one with most potential impact. Successful early identification of p-MCI patients opens up the possibility for improving clinical trials aimed at assessing preventive care treatments. Moradi *et al.* [9] specifically focused on the discrimination of p-MCI vs. s-MCI patients up to 3 years prior to conversion. Tong *et al.* [12] also identified p-MCI subjects depending on their similarity with a pre-defined dictionary containing both HC and AD subjects. This latter work was inspired by an hippocampal grading method by Coupé *et al.* [4] (i.e., SNIPE) that assessed hippocampal abnormality based on local similarities to a pre-defined training library. The grade produced by SNIPE could discriminate s-MCI vs. p-MCI with high accuracy.

The structures in the medial temporal lobe (MTL), including the hippocampus, are among the first ones to be atrophied during the early stages of AD [11]. Strictly speaking, atrophy can only be measured using repeated acquisitions from the same subject over time (rather than using a single MRI, as in the above methods). Several approaches agree in finding atrophy rates in the MTL structures following the trend AD > MCI > HC [2,3]. However, these approaches are not designed for personalized predictions at the individual level and can only reveal the general trends in the population.

We propose a novel method to describe, with a high level of detail, the atrophy patterns across a pair of MRI scans from the same subject at different time points. The proposed descriptor is suitable for being used by machine learning techniques for personalized medicine. Inspired by patch-based label fusion in multi-atlas segmentation [5], our descriptor computes local patch-wise similarities between baseline and follow-up images. Therefore, one-to-many correspondences are used to encode local displacements. For the early prediction of AD, we feed the proposed high-dimensional descriptors extracted from the hippocampal region to a conventional logistic regression classifier.

Other learning-based methods use longitudinal data to predict AD in the first stage of the pathology. Zhu *et al.* [15] proposed a constrained SVM specifically designed for longitudinal data. Jie *et al.* [8] proposed a constrained regression for the prediction of the evolution of cognitive scores in AD patients. The main difference between these methods and the proposed one is that the former ones propose longitudinally-aware classifiers that use conventional MRI images, whereas we propose longitudinally-specific descriptors that can be used by conventional classifiers.

2 Method

We present an atrophy descriptor between a pair of baseline B_i and follow-up F_i images for the i-th patient, aimed at capturing the subtle atrophy patterns discriminating s-MCI and p-MCI patients. In order to bring the pair of images into correspondence while still preserving the local differences due to atrophy, we affinely register the follow-up image to its baseline. We use the notation $F_i^{\to B}$ to denote that the follow-up image has been registered to its corresponding baseline. In the case that we have more than one follow-up image per patient, we can divide the entire sequence into a set of pairs baseline/follow-up and treat them independently. The proposed method is divided in the following steps: (i) defining the region-of-interest (ROI), (ii) computing the patch-based similarity maps, (iii) building the atrophy descriptor and (iv) learning the classifier.

2.1 Region of Interest

We extract the high-dimensional atrophy descriptors from a ROI around the hippocampus. As shown in the literature, the hippocampus is among the first regions to be atrophied due to AD [11] and therefore it is a reasonable choice as ROI for early prediction of AD [5,6]. We propagate the hippocampal ROI, denoted as Ω, from a template image T onto each baseline B_i using spatial warpings $\mathcal{T}_{T \to B_i}$ obtained via non-rigid image registration. The hippocampal ROI in the template was computed by dilating (with a structuring element of $3 \times 3 \times 3$) the hippocampal segmentation obtained through multi-atlas segmentation [5]. Figure 1 shows the hippocampal ROI (in red) overlaid onto the template.

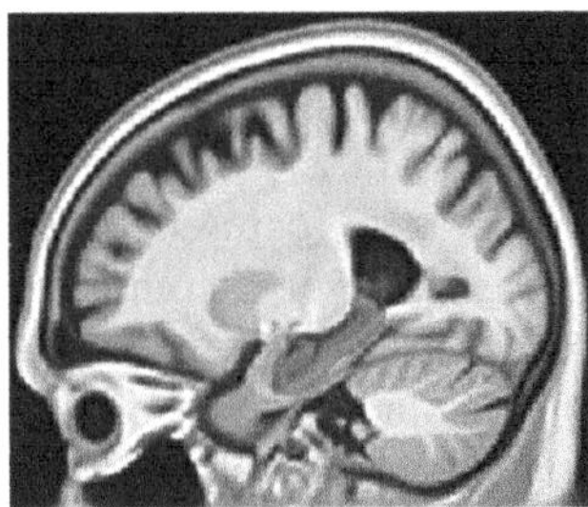

Fig. 1. Hippocampal ROI (in red) overlaid onto a template image. (Color figure online)

Finally, let us denote as $\left(B_i\left(x\right), F_i^{\to B}\left(x\right)\right), x \in \Omega_i$, the pair of voxel intensities at corresponding location x within the ROI Ω_i in the baseline and follow-up images of a given subject.

2.2 Patch-Based Similarity Maps

We encode the atrophy patterns as one-to-many correspondences between each point in the baseline $x \in \Omega_i$ and the neighboring points in the follow-up $x' \in \mathcal{N}_x$, where $\mathcal{N}_x$ is a cubic neighborhood of size s^3 around point x. This gives high-dimensional information about local displacements undergone by each point between the two scans. We use the similarity between image patches to compute the local correspondences, where the patches centered at x and x' in the baseline and follow-up images are defined respectively as $\mathcal{P}_i^B(x), \mathcal{P}_i^F(x')$. In our experiments we use a patch size of $3 \times 3 \times 3$.

For each subject, we compute a set of similarity maps $W_i^{(j)}, j = 1 \ldots s^3$, one for each offset in the cubic neighborhood $\mathcal{N}_x$, as follows:

$$W_i^{(j)}(x) = \exp\left(\frac{-\|\mathcal{P}_i^B(x) - \mathcal{P}_i^F(\mathcal{N}_x(j))\|_2^2}{h^2}\right) \quad (1)$$

where $\mathcal{N}_x(j)$ is the j-th offset in the cubic neighborhood and we use the exponential of the negative sum of squared differences as measure of patch similarity with a normalization constant $h = \sum_j \|\mathcal{P}_i^B(x) - \mathcal{P}_i^F(\mathcal{N}_x(j))\|_2$. Figure 2 shows examples of similarity maps across each neighbor offset in a cubic 27-neighborhood.

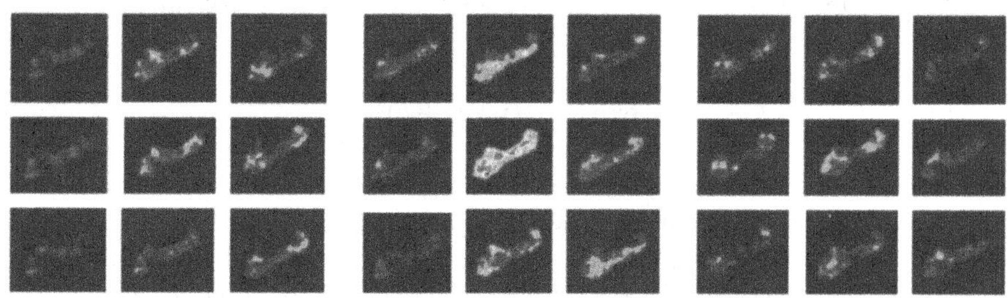

Fig. 2. Each of the 27 tiles shows the similarity map for a different neighbor, with red and blue denoting higher and lower similarities, respectively. We have used a cubic neighborhood of size $s^3 = 3 \times 3 \times 3 = 27$. Tiles in each group of 9 are coherently placed according to their neighborhood offset within the sagittal plane. The three groups correspond to neighbors along the sagittal axis.

2.3 Atrophy Descriptors

The proposed atrophy descriptors are built by encapsulating the similarity maps $W_i^{(j)}$ into feature vectors according to the following steps:

1. We spatially align to a reference space the similarity maps, denoted as $\tilde{W}_i^{(j)}$, using the inverse non-rigid transformations between template and baselines $\mathcal{T}_{T \to B_i}^{-1}$ (recall that similarity maps originally lie in the space of their baseline images).
2. To compensate for moderate registration errors, we smooth the warped similarities using a Gaussian kernel of width σ.
3. We build the longitudinal atrophy descriptor for i-th subject, denoted as $\mathbf{z}_i$, by concatenating the similarities across ROI locations and neighbors, i.e., $\left\{\tilde{W}_i^{(j)}(x) \,|x \in \Omega, j = 1 \ldots s^3\right\}$ (in practice, we subsample the locations with a step size ρ along each dimension in order to reduce redundancy and decrease the vector's length).

The length of the final vector is approximately $|\Omega| \cdot s^3/\rho^3$. In our experiments we set $\sigma = 1.0$, $s^3 = 27$ and $\rho = 2$.

2.4 Learning

Given the atrophy descriptors computed in the previous section in a population of training subjects $\{\mathbf{z}_i, i = 1 \ldots n\}$, we learn a logistic regression classifier to predict the future outcome of each patient, denoted as $y_i = \{-1, 1\}$, for s-MCI and p-MCI, respectively. Prior to learning, we select the most important features by training a random forest classifier with 1000 trees on the future outcome of each patient. As input to the logistic regression classifier, we only use the features with an importance above $0.5 \cdot \mu$, where the importance is computed according how much a feature decreases the average impurity on the forest and μ is the average importance across features[1]. After the feature selection step, we train a logistic regression classifier by minimizing the empirical loss over our training data subject to some regularization constraint. We define the optimization as:

$$\min_{\mathbf{v},b} \sum_{i}^{n} \frac{1}{1 + \exp\left(-y_i \left(\mathbf{v}^\top \mathbf{z}'_i + b\right)\right)} + \lambda \|\mathbf{v}\|_1 , \tag{2}$$

where $\mathbf{v}$ and b are the parameters of the logistic regression classifier and $\mathbf{z}'_i$ is the vector of selected features from the i-th subject. The first term penalizes the classification errors and the second term, modulated by the scalar λ, enforces the sparseness of the coefficients-vector $\mathbf{v}$ through the L_1-norm. The sparsity regularization is suitable when the number of features is much larger than the number of training samples, as in our case. Given the atrophy descriptor extracted from a new testing subject $\mathbf{z}$, first we obtain $\mathbf{z}'$ by picking the most important features as determined during training and then we classify it as p-MCI or s-MCI according to the output of the function: $\text{sign}\left(f\left(\mathbf{z}'; \mathbf{v}, b\right)\right)$, where $f\left(\cdot\right)$ is the learned logistic regression classifier.

3 Experiments

We evaluate our method in classification experiments between MCI patients that remain stable (i.e., s-MCI) and MCI patients that will progress to AD in the following 3 years (i.e., p-MCI). We use the same subset of ADNI[2] as in [9,12], containing 164 p-MCI and 100 s-MCI subjects[3].

We use the first scan (i.e., baseline, B_i) and second scan (i.e., follow-up F_i) of each subject in order to compute the atrophy descriptors. Images are corrected for inhomogeneities with the N4 algorithm [13] and their histograms linearly matched to a reference template [10]. Follow-up images F_i are affinely registered to their respective baselines B_i with ANTs [1]. Subsequently, also with ANTs, we compute non-rigid spatial transformations from the MNI152 template to each of the baselines $\mathcal{T}_{T \rightarrow B_i}$.

---

[1] This is implemented in the `feature_importance_` attribute of the random forest classifier in `scikit-learn` package in Python.

[2] http://www.adni-info.org/.

[3] More details at: https://sites.google.com/site/machinelearning4mcitoad/.

For each subject, we build the atrophy descriptors as follows:

1. The hippocampal ROI is propagated from the template to each of the baselines B_i, as described in Sect. 2.1.
2. Similarity maps $W_i^{(j)}$ are computed using baseline and registered follow-up scans, as described in Sect. 2.2.
3. Atrophy descriptors $\mathbf{z}_i$ are built after smoothing and subsampling the warped similarity maps $\tilde{W}_i^{(j)}$, as described in Sect. 2.3.

Alternatively, we also compute more compact representations by decomposing the similarities at each point through PCA. We took the first 10 components explaining > 90% of the variance of the data.

Table 1 shows the average classification accuracy obtained by logistic regression with the proposed atrophy descriptors in 10-fold cross-validation experiments (with and without PCA decomposition) for a range of regularization strengths λ.

Table 1. Accuracy of the proposed method in 10-fold cross-validation classification of s-MCI and p-MCI subjects for increasing regularization strenghts. First row corresponds to the original proposed descriptor. Second row corresponds to the proposed descriptor with an additional PCA decomposition step.

	$\lambda = 0.1$	$\lambda = 1.0$	$\lambda = 10$	$\lambda = 50$	$\lambda = 100$	$\lambda = 200$	$\lambda = 300$	$\lambda = 500$
Original	0.709	0.744	0.745	0.745	**0.766**	0.757	0.754	0.753
PCA	0.715	0.732	**0.742**	0.737	0.733	0.737	0.713	0.741

As we can see in Table 1, the additional PCA decomposition step degrades the discrimination accuracy, thus suggesting that some important information may be lost after the linear decomposition in the present application. Note that, even we only sacrifice 10% of the variance of the data in the PCA decomposition, we may also lose some structure imposed by the normalization of the similarities (i.e., similarities may not add up to one after the reconstruction).

For comparison, in Table 2 we show the results reported by state-of-the-art methods in s-MCI vs. p-MCI classification using MRI features (including some methods using the same dataset as ours).

Table 2. Perfomance in s-MCI vs. p-MCI classification of state-of-the-art methods using only MRI features. The former 4 methods in the table use only a single baseline MRI for classification whereas the latter 3 use at least one longitudinal follow-up as well. See the main text for details about performances reported as an interval. Methods with an asterisk (*) have been evaluated in the same dataset as the proposed method.

	Cross-sectional				Longitudinal		
Method	Moradi [9]*	Tong [12]*	Coupé [4]	Wolz [14]	Zhu [15]	Jie [8]	Proposed
Perform.	0.747	0.789	0.74	0.68	0.76–0.84	0.757	0.766

Comparing results in Table 2, we can see that our method achieves state-of-the-art performance. Our results are directly comparable to [9,12], since we use the same dataset. It is worth noting that [9,12] use the whole brain whereas we only use the hippocampal ROI. On the other hand, we use a pair of baseline and follow-up scans whereas [9,12] only use single baseline scan for classification. Coupé *et al.* [4] also focused on the hippocampal ROI (including enthorinal cortex), suggesting that this area might convey important information for early AD classification [11]. As another difference, results of [4,14] correspond to early prediction of up to 4 years before conversion, whereas our results (as well as those in [9,12]) correspond to prediction up to 3 years before conversion. The rest of longitudinal methods (i.e., [8,15]) use at least 4 follow-up scans for each subject, whereas we use only 1 baseline and 1 follow-up scan. Zhu *et al.* [15] discriminate between progression to AD at intervals 18, 12, 6 and 0 months with accuracies 0.76, 0.81, 0.83 and 0.84, respectively, hence the interval 0.76–0.84 in the table.

4 Conclusions

We have presented a high-dimensional atrophy descriptor for early AD prediction using longitudinal MRI data. We achieve state-of-the-art performance by feeding our proposed descriptor to a conventional logistic regression classifier. Results suggest that our descriptor is suitable for capturing subtle atrophic patterns distinguishing s-MCI and p-MCI patients up to 3 years before conversion. Indeed, the hippocampal ROI is a suitable region for prediction in the early stages because it is among the first areas revealing atrophy due to AD [11]. Other methods have also focused in this ROI, achieving comparable performance to methods using the whole brain [4]. Effective ways to reduce the dimensionality should be explored in order to extend the use of the proposed descriptor to larger areas of the brain. Results in [15] suggest room for improvement in using the full sequence of follow-up scans (instead of the first 2 ones). Possible lines of future work include combining our descriptor extracted from full follow-up sequences with longitudinally-aware classifiers.

Acknowledgements. The first author is co-financed by the Marie Curie FP7-PEOPLE-2012-COFUND 462 Action. Grant agreement no: 600387.

References

1. Avants, B.B., Epstein, C.L., Grossman, M., Gee, J.C.: Symmetric diffeomorphic image registration with cross-correlation: evaluating automated labeling of elderly and neurodegenerative brain. Med. Image Anal. **12**(1), 26–41 (2008)

2. Cash, D.M., Frost, C., Iheme, L.O., Ünay, D., Kandemir, M., Fripp, J., Salvado, O., Bourgeat, P., Reuter, M., Fischl, B., Lorenzi, M., Frisoni, G.B., Pennec, X., Peirson, R.K., Gunter, J.L., Senjem, M.L., Jack, C.R., Guizard, N., Fonov, V.S., Collins, D.L., Modat, M., Cardoso, M.J., Leung, K.K., Wang, H., Das, S.R., Yushkevich, P.A., Malone, I.B., Fox, N.C., Schott, J.M., Ourselin, S.: Assessing atrophy measurement techniques in dementia: results from the MIRIAD atrophy challenge. NeuroImage **123**, 149–164 (2015)
3. Chincarini, A., Sensi, F., Rei, L., Gemme, G., Squarcia, S., Longo, R., Brun, F., Tangaro, S., Bellotti, R., Amoroso, N., Bocchetta, M., Redolfi, A., Bosco, P., Boccardi, M., Frisoni, G.B., Nobili, F.: Integrating longitudinal information in hippocampal volume measurements for the early detection of Alzheimer's disease. NeuroImage **125**, 834–847 (2016)
4. Coupé, P., Eskildsen, S.F., Manjón, J.V., Fonov, V.S., Pruessner, J.C., Allard, M., Collins, D.L.: Scoring by nonlocal image patch estimator for early detection of Alzheimer's disease. NeuroImage Clin. **1**, 141–152 (2012)
5. Coupé, P., Manjón, J.V., Fonov, V.S., Pruessner, J., Robles, M., Collins, D.L.: Patch-based segmentation using expert priors: application to hippocampus and ventricle segmentation. NeuroImage **54**(2), 940–954 (2011)
6. Cuingnet, R., Gerardin, E., Tessieras, J., Auzias, G., Lehéricy, S., Habert, M.O., Chupin, M., Benali, H., Colliot, O.: Automatic classification of patients with Alzheimer's disease from structural MRI: a comparison of ten methods using the ADNI database. NeuroImage **56**, 766–781 (2011)
7. Frisoni, G.B., Fox, N.C., Jack, C.R., Scheltens, P., Thompson, P.M.: The clinical use of structural MRI in Alzheimer disease. Nat. Rev. Neurol. **6**(2), 67–77 (2010)
8. Jie, B., Liu, M., Zhang, D., Shen, D.: Temporally-constrained group sparse learning for longitudinal data analysis in Alzheimer's disease. IEEE Trans. Biomed. Eng. **64**(1), 238–249 (2015)
9. Moradi, E., Pepe, A., Gaser, C., Huttunen, H., Tohka, J.: Machine learning framework for early MRI-based Alzheimer's conversion prediction in MCI subjects. NeuroImage **104**, 398–412 (2015)
10. Nyúl, L.G., Udupa, J.K.: On standardizing the mr image instensity scale. Magn. Reson. Med. **42**(6), 1072–1081 (1999)
11. Thompson, P.M., Hayashi, K.M., de Zubicaray, G., Janke, A.L., Rose, S.E., Semple, J., Herman, D., Hong, M.S., Dittmer, S.S., Doddrell, D.M., Toga, A.W.: Dynamics of gray matter loss in Alzheimer's disease. J. Neurosci. **23**(3), 994–1005 (2003)
12. Tong, T., Gao, Q., Guerrero, R., Ledig, C., Chen, L., Rueckert, D.: A Novel grading biomarker for the prediction of conversion from Mild cognitive impairment to Alzheimer's disease. IEEE Trans. Biomed. Eng. **64**(1), 155–165 (2017)
13. Tustison, N.J., Avants, B.B., Cook, P.A., Zheng, Y., Egan, A., Yushkevich, P.A., Gee, J.C.: N4ITK: improved N3 bias correction. IEEE Trans. Med. Imaging **29**(6), 1310–1320 (2010)
14. Wolz, R., Julkunen, V., Koikkalainen, J., Niskanen, E., Zhang, D.P., Rueckert, D., Soininen, H., Lötjönen, J.: Multi-method analysis of MRI images in early diagnostics of Alzheimer's disease. PLOS ONE **6**, 10 (2011)
15. Zhu, Y., Zhu, X., Kim, M., Shen, D., Wu, G.: Early diagnosis of Alzheimer's disease by joint feature selection and classification on temporally structured support vector machine. In: MICCAI (2016)

Adaptive Fusion of Texture-Based Grading: Application to Alzheimer's Disease Detection

Kilian Hett[1,2(✉)], Vinh-Thong Ta[1,2,3], José V. Manjón[4], Pierrick Coupé[1,2], and the Alzheimer's Disease Neuroimaging Initiative

[1] Univ. Bordeaux, LaBRI, UMR 5800, PICTURA, 33400 Talence, France
kilian.hett@labri.fr
[2] CNRS, LaBRI, UMR 5800, PICTURA, 33400 Talence, France
[3] Bordeaux INP, LaBRI, UMR 5800, PICTURA, 33600 Pessac, France
[4] ITACA, Universitat Politècnia de València, 46022 Valencia, Spain

Abstract. Alzheimer's disease is a neurodegenerative process leading to irreversible mental dysfunctions. The development of new biomarkers is crucial to perform an early detection of this disease. Among new biomarkers proposed during the last decades, patch-based grading framework demonstrated state-of-the-art results. In this paper, we study the potential using texture information based on Gabor filters to improve patch-based grading method performance, with a focus on the hippocampal structure. We also propose a novel fusion framework to efficiently combine multiple grading maps derived from a Gabor filters bank. Finally, we compare our new texture-based grading biomarker with the state-of-the-art approaches to demonstrate the high potential of the proposed method.

Keywords: Patch-based grading fusion · Multi-features · Alzheimer's disease classification · Mild Cognitive Impairment

1 Introduction

Alzheimer's disease (AD) is the most prevalent dementia. AD is characterized by an irreversible neurodegeneration leading to mental dysfunctions. Subjects with Mild Cognitive Impairment (MCI) present higher risk to develop AD. To date, diagnosis of AD is established after advanced brain structure alterations motivating the crucial need to develop new imaging biomarkers able to detect the early stages of the disease. Furthermore, the early detection of AD can accelerate the development of new therapies by making easier the design of clinical trials.

Data used in preparation of this article were obtained from the Alzheimer's Disease Neuroimaging Initiative (ADNI) database (adni.loni.usc.edu). As such, the investigators within the ADNI contributed to the design and implementation of ADNI and/or provided data but did not participate in analysis or writing of this report. A complete listing of ADNI investigators can be found at: http://adni.loni.usc.edu/wp-content/uploads/how_to_apply/ADNI_Acknowledgement_List.pdf.

© Springer International Publishing AG 2017
G. Wu et al. (Eds.): Patch-MI 2017, LNCS 10530, pp. 82–89, 2017.
DOI: 10.1007/978-3-319-67434-6_10

During the last decades, new biomarkers with competitive performances were developed to detect AD by taking advantage of the improvement of medical imaging like magnetic resonance imaging (MRI) [1].

Most of the proposed methods have been based on specific regions of interest (ROI). Among structures impacted by AD, previous investigations mainly focused on medial temporal lobe and especially on hippocampus (HC). Alterations on this structure are usually estimated using volume, shape or cortical thickness measurements [11]. Besides ROI-based methods, whole brain analyses performed on structural MRI (s-MRI) have also been proposed to detect areas impacted by AD. These methods are usually based on voxel-based morphometry (VBM) or tensor based morphometry (TBM) frameworks. It is interesting to note that both VBM and ROI-based studies confirmed that medial temporal lobe is a key area to detect the first signs of AD [11]. In the medial temporal lobe, the HC is one of the earliest region altered by AD. Recently, advanced methods were proposed to capture structural alterations of HC. Those techniques demonstrated their efficiency to detect the different stages of AD [8]. Among them, patch-based methods obtained competitive results to detect the earliest stages of AD [2,7,9]. Therefore, such advanced image analysis methods seem promising candidates to perform AD tracking. Recently, [4] demonstrated the efficiency of using edge detection filters to improve of patch-based segmentation. This result highlights that patches comparison can be improved by estimating patterns similarity on derivative image features. Moreover, it has been recently showed that HC texture plays a crucial role for the detection of early stages of AD [8]. Therefore, we propose to perform patch-based grading on multiple texture maps obtained with Gabor filters. Gabor filters are designed to detect salient features at specific resolution and direction. These filters were widely used for texture classification [13]. Consequently, the proposed strategy enables at the same time to improve patches comparison and to capture HC texture modifications occurring at the first stages of the pathology.

Contributions: The first contribution of this work is intended to develop a new texture-based grading framework to better capture structural alterations caused by AD. Secondly, in order to combine all the grading maps estimated on texture maps, we propose an innovate adaptive fusion strategy based on local confidence criterion. This fusion framework can be applied to any patch-based processing to combine different features or modalities. Moreover, contrary to usual grading-based methods, we propose a classification step involving weak classifiers distribution to better discriminate pathologies stages. Finally, to highlight the improvement of classification performances provided by our new framework, we compare our new biomarker with the state-of-the-art biomarkers and demonstrate its efficiency.

2 Materials and Methods

2.1 Dataset

Data used in this work were obtained from Alzheimer's Disease Neuroimaging Initiative (ADNI) dataset[1]. ADNI is a North American campaign launched in 2003 with aims to provide MRI, positron emission tomography scans, clinical neurological measures and other biomarkers. The data used in this study are all the baseline T1-weighted (T1-w) MRI of the ADNI1 phase. This dataset includes AD patients, MCI and cognitive normal (CN) subjects. The group of MCI is composed of subjects who have abnormal memory dysfunctions and embed two groups, the first one is composed with patients having stable MCI (sMCI) and the second one is composed with patients with progressive MCI (pMCI). The information of the dataset used in our work is summarized in Table 1.

Table 1. Description of the dataset used in this work. Data are provided by ADNI.

Characteristic/group	CN	sMCI	pMCI	AD
Number of subjects	226	223	165	186
Ages (years)	76.0 ± 5.0	75.1 ± 7.5	74.5 ± 7.2	75.3 ± 7.4
Sex (M/F)	117/109	150/73	101/64	98/88
MMSE	29.05 ± 0.9	27.1 ± 2.5	26.3 ± 2.0	22.8 ± 2.9

2.2 Preprocessing

All the T1-w images were processed using the volBrain system [12][2]. This system is based on an advanced pipeline providing automatic segmentation of different brain structures from T1-w MRI. The preprocessing is based on: (a) a denoising step with an adaptive non-local means filter, (b) an affine registration in the MNI space, (c) a correction of the image inhomogeneities and (d) an intensity normalization.

2.3 Methods

Patch-Based Grading: Grading framework uses patch-based techniques to capture modifications related to anatomical degradations caused by AD [2]. To date, patch-based grading methods demonstrate state-of-the-art performances to detect the earliest stages of AD [6,10]. To determine the pathological status of a subject, grading-based methods estimate at each voxel the state of cerebral tissues using anatomical patterns extracted from a training library T composed of two datasets, one with images from CN subjects and one with AD patients. Then, for each voxel of the considered subject, the patch-based grading method

[1] http://adni.loni.ucla.edu.

[2] http://volbrain.upv.es.

produces a weak classifier denoted g. This weak classifier is based on the similarity between the patch surrounding the voxel under study x_i and a set K_i of similar patches extracted from T. In this work, we used an approximative nearest neighbor method to drastically reduce the required computational time [5]. The grading value g at x_i is defined as:

$$g(x_i) = \frac{\sum_{x_{j,t} \in K_i} w(x_i, x_{j,t}) p_t}{\sum_{x_{j,t} \in K_i} w(x_i, x_{j,t})} \tag{1}$$

where $x_{j,t}$ is the voxel j belonging to the training template $t \in T$. $w(x_i, x_{j,t})$ is the weight assigned to the pathological status p_t of t. We estimate w such as:

$$w(x_i, x_{j,t}) = e^{1 - \frac{(d(x_i, x_{j,t}))^2}{h^2 + \epsilon}} \tag{2}$$

where $h = \min_{x_{j,t}} d(x_i, x_{j,t})$ with $\epsilon \to 0$, d is a distance between two patches surrounding the voxels x_i and $x_{j,t}$. p_t is set to -1 for patches extracted from AD patient and to 1 for those extracted from CN subject. The L2-norm is used to estimate the similarly between patches. Thus, our patch-based grading method provides at each voxel a score representing an estimation of the alterations caused by AD.

Texture Maps Estimation: The estimation of patch similarities could be improved by using texture representation instead of using raw intensities. Indeed, it was demonstrated that the use of edge detectors improves patch-based segmentation accuracy [4]. Moreover, it was also demonstrated that HC textural information plays an important role in AD detection [8]. Hence, we propose a new texture-based grading framework that simultaneously captures HC texture alterations and improves patches similarity estimation. In this work, texture information is extracted from MRI using a bank of 3D Gabor filters. We used Gabor filters since they are designed to detect texture patterns at different scales and directions [13]. In the proposed pipeline (see Fig. 1), the preprocessed MRI of the subject under study is filtered with a bank of Gabor filters to obtain multiple texture maps. It has to be noted that all the training library is also filtered with the same filters bank. Therefore, for each texture map, a texture-based grading map can be estimated.

Adaptive Fusion: In this work, we propose an novel framework to fuse the multiple texture-based grading maps obtained from the estimated texture maps. Our fusion strategy is based on the fact that all the estimated grading maps may not have the same relevance, but more importantly all local weak classifiers in these maps do not have the same quality. Hence, at each location, we propose to combine weak classifiers derived from multiple texture maps according to a confidence criterion. Therefore, the grading value of a texture-based grading map m, denoted g_m, at voxel x_i, is weighted by $\alpha_m(x_i) = \sum_{x_{j,t} \in K_{i,m}} w_m(x_i, x_{j,t})$ that reflects the confidence of g_m. Thus, each texture-based grading map provides a weak classifier at each voxel that is weighted with its degree of confidence $\alpha_m(x_i)$. At the end, the final grading value, denoted g_M, resulting from our adaptive fusion strategy is given by;

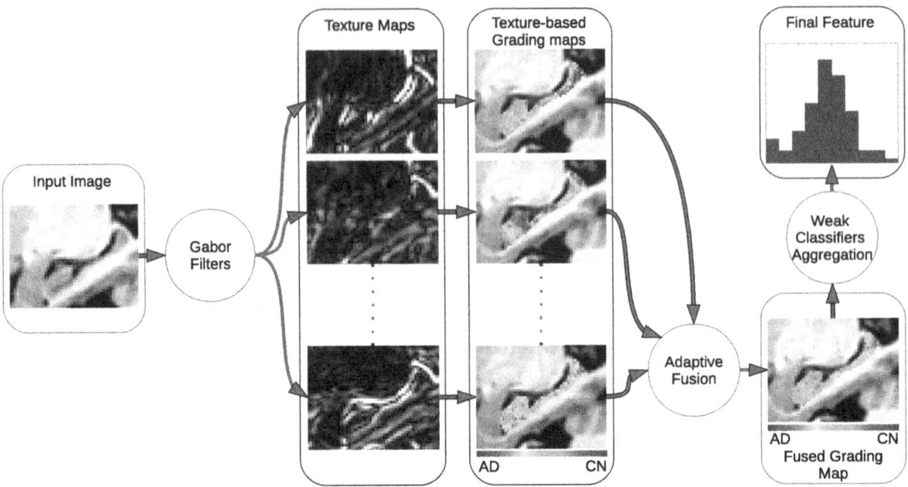

Fig. 1. Proposed adaptive fusion of texture-based grading framework.: from left to right, the T1-w input data, the texture maps for different directions, the intermediate texture-based grading maps, the final fused grading map and the histogram-based weak classifiers aggregation.

$$g_M(x_i) = \frac{\sum_{m \in M} \alpha_m(x_i) g_m(x_i)}{\sum_{m \in M} \alpha_m(x_i)} . \tag{3}$$

The proposed fusion framework is spatially adaptive and take advantage of having access to a local degree of confidence $\alpha_m(x_i)$ for each grading map m. Basically, the confidence $\alpha_m(x_i)$ gives more weight to a weak classifier estimated with a well matched set of patches. Our adaptive fusion strategy can applied to any patch-based processing to combine multiple feature or modalities.

Weak Classifiers Aggregation: First, to prevent bias introduced by structure alterations related to aging, all the grading values are age corrected with a linear regression based on the CN group [3]. In previous works on patch-based grading [2,5], the weak classifier aggregation was performed using a simple averaging. While using a strategy based on averaging enables to be robust to noise, this may remove relevant information on weak classifiers distribution. Therefore, in this paper we propose to approximate weak classifiers distribution using histogram. Consequently, we classify histogram bins instead of classifying mean grading value over the segmentation mask. Here, histograms were separately estimated for right and left hippocampus.

Validation: During our experiments, texture maps were obtained using one scale and 3 orthogonal directions. The texture-based grading maps were estimated using patches of $5 \times 5 \times 5$ voxels. The grading step based on an optimized PatchMatch [5] was performed using $K = 50$. The required computational time was 3 s per texture maps, thus the global grading step required 10 s with our setup. Our new texture-based grading framework was validated with a leave-one-out cross validation procedure. A support vector machine (SVM) was used to classify each test subject. The results of each experiment were compared in terms of accuracy (ACC) and area under the ROC curve (AUC). The AUC is estimated with the *a posteriori* probabilities provided by the SVM classifier. We carried out several experiments: CN vs. AD, CN vs. pMCI, AD vs. sMCI and sMCI vs. pMCI.

3 Results

Firstly, in order to validate the improvement provided by our method, we compare results obtained with our framework using raw intensities (T1-w grading) and texture maps. T1-w and texture-based grading were estimated using exactly the same pipeline involving adaptive fusion and histogram-based weak classifiers aggregation. Table 2 summarizes the results of T1-w grading and our proposed method. Results are expressed with area under the curve (AUC) measure. As it is shown, texture-based grading improves classification performances in all experiments especially MCI classification with 94.2% of AUC in CN vs. AD, 90.9% of AUC in the CN vs. pMCI, 81.3% of AUC in AD vs. sMCI and 75.4% of AUC in sMCI vs. pMCI comparisons. During our experiments, weak classifiers aggregation based on histogram did not provide improvement in CN vs. AD comparison. That could be explained by the fact that CN and AD distributions are separated. However, in sMCI vs. pMCI case, the two distributions are less separable and histogram representation yielded to better classification performances. The experiments carried out showed that the use of only one scale is enough. Moreover, using more than 3 directions did not improve the results while increasing computational time.

Table 3 summarizes the comparison of our proposed method with other grading methods proposed in the literature. In addition, classification results obtained with Deep Learning (DL) [14] ensemble are provided for comparison with last advanced methods. The results on Table 3 are expressed in accuracy (ACC). First, to compare classification results using the same structure, the proposed framework is compared with grading methods based on HC (see the upper part of Table 3). This comparison shows that our method provides the best results among HC-based grading methods. It reaches 91.3% of ACC for CN vs. AD, and 71.1% of ACC for sMCI vs. pMCI comparisons. These results demonstrate that texture maps provide valuable information during the grading process. At the lower part of Table 3, we compare the performance of our HC-based grading method with those using the whole brain.

Table 2. Comparison of different features HC-based, all results are expressed in AUC.

Features	CN vs. AD (AUC in %)	CN vs. pMCI (AUC in %)	AD vs. sMCI (AUC in %)	sMCI vs. pMCI (AUC in %)
T1-w grading	93.5	90.0	81.1	73.6
Proposed method	**94.2**	**90.9**	**81.3**	**75.4**

First, for AD vs. CN, the proposed method obtained similar or better results than those using whole brain and requiring non linear registration [7] while our method only requires affine registration and proposes a fast grading step (i.e., 10 s). Second, for sMCI vs. pMCI, our method obtained better results than all the methods involving a simple affine registration [10]. On the other hand, the best results for sMCI vs. pMCI are produced by whole brain grading [6,10] using non linear registration. The improvement when using non linear registration is observed for HC-based and whole brain methods [10]. However, this improvement is obtained at the expense of using non linear registration, which is subject to failure and requires high computational time. Finally, our method also demonstrated competitive performances for AD vs. CN classification compared to the most advanced DL methods using whole brain and non linear registration. In addition, this comparison shows that patch-based grading methods [6,10] obtain similar or better results than recent DL methods [14] when applied with similar settings.

To conclude, according to our comparison, whole brain methods enable a better classification of sMCI vs. pMCI. Hence, in further works, we will investigate the extension of our texture-based grading framework to whole brain analysis.

Table 3. Comparison with state-of-the-art methods, all the results are expressed in accuracy.

Methods	Registration	Features	CN vs. AD (ACC in %)	sMCI vs. pMCI (ACC in %)
Hippocampus				
Original grading [2]	Affine	Intensity	88.0	71.0
Multiple instance grading [9]	Affine	Intensity	89.0	70.0
Sparse-based grading [10]	Affine	Intensity	–	66.0
Sparse-based grading [10]	Non linear	Intensity	–	69.0
Proposed method	Affine	Texture	**91.3**	**71.1**
Whole brain				
Ensemble grading [6]	Non linear	GM Map	–	**75.6**
Sparse-based grading [10]	Affine	Intensity	–	66.7
Sparse-based grading [10]	Non linear	Intensity	–	75.0
Sparse ensemble grading [7]	Non linear	GM Map	90.8	–
Deep ensemble learning [14]	Non linear	GM Map	91.0	74.8

4 Conclusion

In this work we propose a new texture-based grading framework to better capture structural alterations caused by AD. Moreover, to combine grading maps estimated on texture maps, we present a new adaptive fusion scheme. We also propose an histogram-based weak classifiers aggregation step to better discriminate early stages of AD. Finally, we demonstrate the competitive performances of our new texture-based grading framework compared to several state-of-the-art biomarkers. In future works, we will investigate the extension of our texture-based grading framework to whole brain analysis.

5 Acknowledgement

This study has been carried out with financial support from the French State, managed by the French National Research Agency (ANR) in the frame of the Investments for the future Program IdEx Bordeaux (ANR-10-IDEX-03-02), Cluster of excellence CPU and TRAIL (HL-MRI ANR-10-LABX-57).

References

1. Bron, E.E., et al.: Standardized evaluation of algorithms for computer-aided diagnosis of dementia based on structural MRI: the CADDementia challenge. NeuroImage **111**, 562–579 (2015)
2. Coupé, P., et al.: Scoring by nonlocal image patch estimator for early detection of Alzheimer's disease. NeuroImage: clin. **1**(1), 141–152 (2012)
3. Dukart, J., et al.: Age correction in dementia-matching to a healthy brain. PLoS One **6**(7), e22193 (2011)
4. Giraud, R., et al.: An optimized patchmatch for multi-scale and multi-feature label fusion. NeuroImage **124**, 770–782 (2016)
5. Hett, K., et al.: Patch-based DTI grading: application to Alzheimer's disease classification. In: Wu, G., Coupé, P., Zhan, Y., Munsell, B.C., Rueckert, D. (eds.) Patch-MI 2016. LNCS, vol. 9993, pp. 76–83. Springer, Cham (2016). doi:10.1007/978-3-319-47118-1_10
6. Komlagan, M., et al.: Anatomically constrained weak classifier fusion for early detection of Alzheimer's disease. In: Wu, G., Zhang, D., Zhou, L. (eds.) MLMI 2014. LNCS, vol. 8679, pp. 141–148. Springer, Cham (2014). doi:10.1007/978-3-319-10581-9_18
7. Liu, M., et al.: Ensemble sparse classification of Alzheimer's disease. NeuroImage **60**(2), 1106–1116 (2012)
8. Sørensen, L., et al.: Differential diagnosis of mild cognitive impairment and Alzheimer's disease using structural MRI cortical thickness, hippocampal shape, hippocampal texture, and volumetry. NeuroImage: Clin. **13**, 470–482 (2016)
9. Tong, T., et al.: Multiple instance learning for classification of dementia in brain MRI. Med. Image Anal. **18**(5), 808–818 (2014)
10. Tong, T., et al.: A novel grading biomarker for the prediction of conversion from mild cognitive impairment to Alzheimer's disease. IEEE Trans. Biomed. Eng. **64**(1), 155–165 (2017)
11. Wolz, R., et al.: Multi-method analysis of MRI images in early diagnostics of Alzheimer's disease. PLoS One **6**(10), e25446 (2011)
12. Manjón, J.V., Coupé, P.: volBrain: an online MRI brain volumetry system. Front. neuroinformatics, 10, 2016
13. Manjunath, B.S., et al.: Texture features for browsing and retrieval of image data. IEEE Trans. Pattern Anal. Mach. Intell. **18**(8), 837–842 (1996)
14. Suk, H.I., et al.: Deep ensemble learning of sparse regression models for brain disease diagnosis. Med. Image Anal. **37**, 101–113 (2017)

Reconstruction, Denoising, Super-Resolution

Micro-CT Guided 3D Reconstruction of Histological Images

Kai Nagara[1(✉)], Holger R. Roth[2], Shota Nakamura[3], Hirohisa Oda[1], Takayasu Moriya[2], Masahiro Oda[2], and Kensaku Mori[2]

[1] Graduate School of Information Science, Nagoya University, Nagoya, Japan
knagara@mori.m.is.nagoya-u.ac.jp

[2] Graduate School of Informatics, Nagoya University, Nagoya, Japan

[3] Graduate School of Medicine, Nagoya University, Nagoya, Japan

Abstract. Histological images are very important for diagnosis of cancer and other diseases. However, during the preparation of the histological slides for microscopy, the 3D information of the tissue specimen gets lost. Therefore, many 3D reconstruction methods for histological images have been proposed. However, most approaches rely on the histological 2D images alone, which makes 3D reconstruction difficult due to the large deformations introduced by cutting and preparing the histological slides. In this work, we propose an image-guided approach to 3D reconstruction of histological images. Before histological preparation of the slides, the specimen is imaged using X-ray microtomography (micro CT). We can then align each histological image back to the micro CT image utilizing non-rigid registration. Our registration results show that our method can provide smooth 3D reconstructions with micro CT guidance.

Keywords: Micro CT · Histological image · 3D reconstruction · Feature matching · Registration

1 Introduction

Histological imaging is important for clinical diagnosis. However, the preparation of microscopic slides requires the cutting of tissue samples into separate 2D slices and the 3D information of the tissue specimen gets lost. The deformations introduced by cutting make 3D reconstruction of histological images difficult based on the histological images alone. Especially, specimens of lung tissue from partial pneumonectomy are difficult to align because of the large flexibility of the tissue.

In this work, we propose an image-guided approach to 3D reconstruction of histological images. Before histological preparation of the slides, the specimen is imaged using X-ray microtomography (μCT). We can then align each histological image back to its original 3D location using non-rigid image registration.

Various methods have been proposed for correlating histological images with 3D imaging modalities [1–6]. Most of these methods have focused on aligning

© Springer International Publishing AG 2017
G. Wu et al. (Eds.): Patch-MI 2017, LNCS 10530, pp. 93–101, 2017.
DOI: 10.1007/978-3-319-67434-6_11

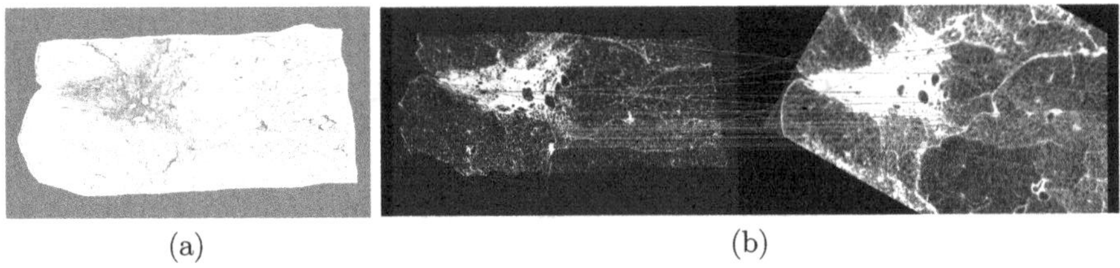

(a) (b)

Fig. 1. A example slice of micro CT volume and histological image. (a) Original histological image, (b) the matching result of glayscaled histological image and micro CT volume. Color points indicate matched feature points (color figure online).

brain images, where there is still significant coherence between the main brain tissue types (white matter, gray matter and cerebrospinal fluid) observable within the histological images. This coherence allows for registration methods that utilize segmentations or histogram matching between the images [1]. Deformable registration of ex vivo MRI to histology imaging was investigated for prostate cancer using both segmentation-based and intensity-based approaches [2]. Dense patch-based methods for correlating tumor histology of rectal cancer and ex vivo MRI were studied in [3]. Similarly, registration of μCT to histology has been studied [4]. However, alignment was only performed rigidly and was constrained to localization of individual 2D histology slices within the 3D μCT volume.

In contrast, we will perform a dense 3D reconstruction of a whole stack of histological images and at the same time correlate them with μCT.

2 Micro-CT Guided 3D Reconstruction

2.1 Method Overview

As a first step, we align the orientation of the histological images in the stack itself. This is done using feature point matching between neighboring slides. Even if there is a deformed slide, the rough overall orientation can be correctly aligned by affine transformations.

Next, each histology slice I_n is registered to the μCT volume V. Again feature point matching is performed between each histological image and each slice of the μCT volume in order to estimate a rigid transformation from the histological image to the μCT images. Finally, non-rigid registration is performed in a slice-by-slice manner between all I_n and V_n in order to recover the finer deformations and produce a 3D reconstruction of the histological image stack.

2.2 Histological Image Alignment

Since the orientation of each histological image is initially arbitrary, feature point matching is performed to align them coherently. However, instead of straightforward matching between adjacent slides, we perform matching within a neighborhood of N slides. This allows us to select the transformation matrix with the most matched feature points within N (Fig. 2).

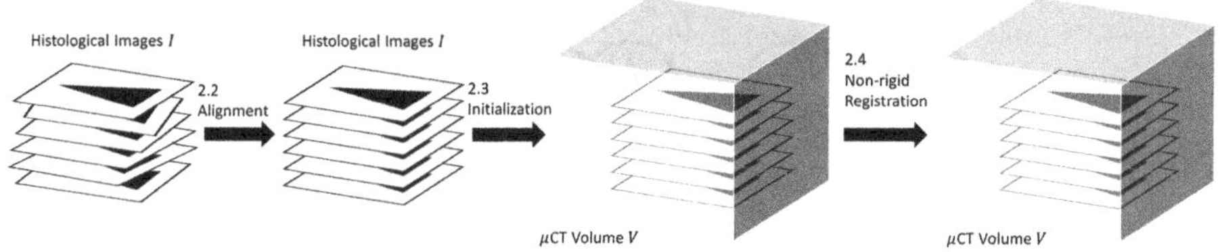

Fig. 2. Outline of reconstruction process. First, we align the orientation of the histological images and register each histological slice to the μCT volume. Finally, non-rigid registration is performed in a slice-by-slice manner between all histological images and μCT volume.

In previous studies [5,6] registration is only performed among directly adjacent slides and the transformation matrices are combined in order to align each slide to a common space. This will encourage the propagation of errors through the slices. Any mistake in registration will be enhanced in subsequent slides and result in incorrect alignments. This accumulation of errors may cause the last slice to deviate greatly with respect to the first slide of the stack.

On the other hand, by using the matching result with the preceding N slices as proposed here, it becomes possible to perform registration while avoiding large incorrect misalignments of the images. In our experiments, we found $N = 10$ to work well.

Feature Matching: For feature point detection and feature description, we use AKAZE [7] which exploits the nonlinear scale spaces of the images based on fast explicit diffusion (FED). AKAZE is implemented in a pyramidal framework and results in a high number of feature points. In comparison to the classical SIFT feature descriptor, AKAZE has been shown to be faster and more robust to rotation [7]. An example of feature matches between histology and μCT is shown in Fig. 1.

First, we detect feature points in all histological images and generate feature descriptors for each point[1]. Next, for each slice, feature point matching between points is performed within all the preceding N slices in a symmetric manner. The images are then transformed using the resulting affine transformation matrices $T_H^{n,0}$ estimated from the pair of images with the most feature matches. That is,

$$T_H^{n,0} = T_H^{l,0} \circ T_H^{n,l}, \tag{1}$$

with

$$l = n - \mathop{\arg\max}_{0<i<N} (\mathrm{MP}(I_n, I_{n-i}) + \mathrm{MP}(I_{n-i}, I_n)). \tag{2}$$

Here, $\mathrm{MP}(I_i, I_j)$ represents the number of matching feature points of image I_i from image I_j computed in both directions. When matching, we apply random

[1] We utilize the OpenCV 3.1.0 implementation http://docs.opencv.org/3.1.0/d8/d30/classcv_1_1AKAZE.html.

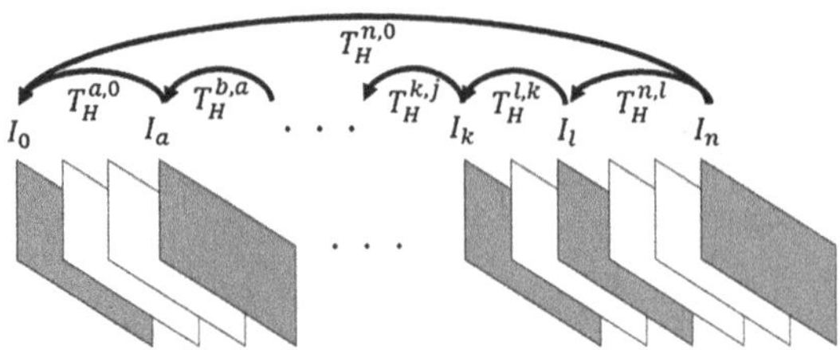

Fig. 3. Feature-based alignment and composition of transformation matrices $T_H^{n,0}$ in order to align each image I_n to the common space of the target image I_0.

sample consensus (RANSAC) for robust estimation of the transformation matrices $T_H^{n,0}$. The resulting transformation matrices are then composed in order to align each slice to the common space of the target image I_0 as shown in Fig. 3.

2.3 Histology to μCT Initialization

The cutting plane of the specimen is marked on μCT before preparation of the histological slices by the performing clinician. Hence, we can use this information to resample the μCT volume V in order to align the histological images I_n to the cross sections V_n. For each slice of the histological image, feature point matching is performed for each slice of the μCT image for initialization. Again, AKAZE is used for feature point detection and matching as in Sect. 2.2. Using this matched set of feature points, RANSAC estimates the transformation matrix between the μCT images and histological images. The parameters estimated here are the scale in xy-direction s_{xy}, the scale in z-direction s_z, the rotation θ around the center of the z-axis, and the translation in three axes $\{t_x, t_y, t_z\}$. Here, the scales in xy-direction and in z-direction are computed separately in order to adjust for the different slice thickness of histological images and μCT .

$$T_V = \begin{pmatrix} s_{xy}\cos\theta & -\sin\theta & 0 & t_x \\ \sin\theta & s_{xy}\cos\theta & 0 & t_y \\ 0 & 0 & s_z & t_z \\ 0 & 0 & 0 & 1 \end{pmatrix} \tag{3}$$

2.4 Slice-by-Slice Non-rigid Registration

Now, each pair of slices of the initialized histological image I_n and μCT volume V_n is aligned using two-dimensional non-rigid registration. For this step we employ an optimization algorithm that formulates the non-rigid registration task as a discrete Markov random field (MRF) [8,9]. In our case, a pairwise non-rigid registration of each 2D slice $I_n, V_n : \in \Omega \subset \mathbb{R}^2$ is performed in order to find the transformation $T : \mathbb{R}^2 \mapsto \mathbb{R}^2$ that maps I_n to V_n. We choose I_n to be the moving image and V_n the target. In non-rigid image registration, the transformation can be defined as

$$T(x) = x + D(x), \tag{4}$$

where $x \in \Omega$ is a point in the image domain and $D(x)$ is a two-dimensional displacement field. The problem of this slice-wise registration is to find the optimal transformation given two images I_n and V_n:

$$\hat{T}_D^n = \arg\min_{T_D^n} \left(\mathcal{E}((T_D^n \circ T_H^{n,0}) I_n, (T_V V)_n) \right), \tag{5}$$

where $\hat{T}_D^n$ is the optimal transformation at the minimum of the objective function $\mathcal{E}$ [8]. Here, $\mathcal{E}$ is composed of a matching term $\mathcal{M}$ and a regularizer $\mathcal{R}$. We utilize normalized cross-correlation (NCC) as the similarity measure $\mathcal{M}$. The regularization $\mathcal{R}$ will be imposed by the MRF formulation itself. In this case, minimizing the energy of an MRF with unary potentials $\bar{\mathbf{g}} = \bar{g}_p(\cdot)$ and pairwise potentials $\bar{\mathbf{f}} = \bar{f}_{pq}(\cdot,\cdot)$ amounts to solving the problem

$$\mathrm{MRF}(\bar{\mathbf{g}}, \bar{\mathbf{f}}) = \min_u \sum_{p \in V} \bar{g}_p(u_p) + \sum_{(p,q) \in V} \bar{f}_p q(u_p, u_q), \tag{6}$$

where each random variable u_p takes values in a discrete label set L, and V and E denote, respectively, the vertices and edges of a MRF graph $G = (V, E)$. In practice, the unary potentials $\bar{g}_p(u_p)$ are typically used for encoding the deformation, whereas the pairwise potentials $\bar{f}_{pq}(u_p, u_q)$ typically act as regularizers and thus play an important role in obtaining high-quality results. In order to optimize the MRF energy for image registration, the Fast-PD solver is used [9]. The utilized implementation[2] considers (free-form deformation) FFDs [10] with cubic B-spline basis functions and control points uniformly distributed over the image domain as the non-rigid transformation model. We employ a common hierarchical coarse-to-fine strategy where the resolution of both the images and the FFD control grid is subsequently refined during the registration process. For registration, we use a Gaussian image pyramid with a standard deviation of 1 and 5 levels. At each level the image dimensions are reduced by a scale factor of 2. In order to control the maximum amount of deformation imposed by the registration, we set an initial control point spacing of 9.5 mm. Which each increasing image resolution in the pyramid, the FFD grid spacing is halved by inserting new control points. This type of image registration approach allows us to first capture the larger deformations and then to focus on the smaller, more subtle details in later iterations as in [8].

3 Results

3.1 Datasets

Two lung specimens were fixed following the Heintzmann method in order to enable high-resolution imaging by μCT (Shimadzu Co., inspeXio SMX-90CT

[2] Drop Version 1.06 http://mrf-registration.net/.

Plus MICRO FOCUS X-RAY CT SYSTEM). The images were acquired with a tube voltage of 90 kV and a tube current of 110 μA. For microscopic imaging the specimen is sliced with a 3 μm thickness before standard H&E staining. After staining a microscopic image is recorded. The original histological image is very large with around $200,000 \times 100,000$ pixels. Therefore, we shrink the images by a factor of 100. The imaging specifications of both μCT and histological images are summarized in Table 1.

Table 1. Specifications

Specifications		Size (pixels)	Resolution (μm)	Number of slices
Case 1	Histological images	1949×1115	22×22	70
	μCT volume	1024×1024	$49 \times 49 \times 49$	1077
Case 2	Histological images	2097×1093	22×22	100
	μCT volume	1024×1024	$52 \times 52 \times 52$	545

3.2 Qualitative Evaluation

For visualization, intensity normalization is performed using histogram matching in order to reduce the difference in density values of each slice. Figure 4 shows an example of the non-rigid registration result. A volume rendering of the 3D reconstruction and the corresponding region in the μCT volume is shown in Fig. 5, in which we can observe vessel-like structures. A more detailed structure can be observed in the proposed histological 3D reconstruction (Fig. 5a) than in μCT (Fig. 5b).

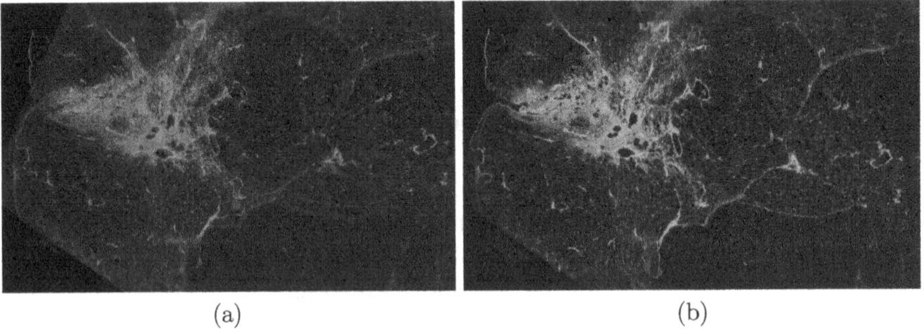

(a) (b)

Fig. 4. A slice of non-rigid registration result. Histological image is shown in green and μCT is shown in red. (a) is before and (b) is after non-rigid registration (Color figure online).

3.3 Quantitative Evaluation

We manually extracted the bronchial regions from the μCT volumes and histological images in order evaluate our methods using the following metrics: Dice index, Jaccard index, recall, and NCC. Figure 6 shows the extracted region in histological images and μCT volume before and after the final 3D reconstruction. The resulting metric scores are shown in Table 2. After the final 3D reconstruction step, all scores of similarity metrics are increased significantly.

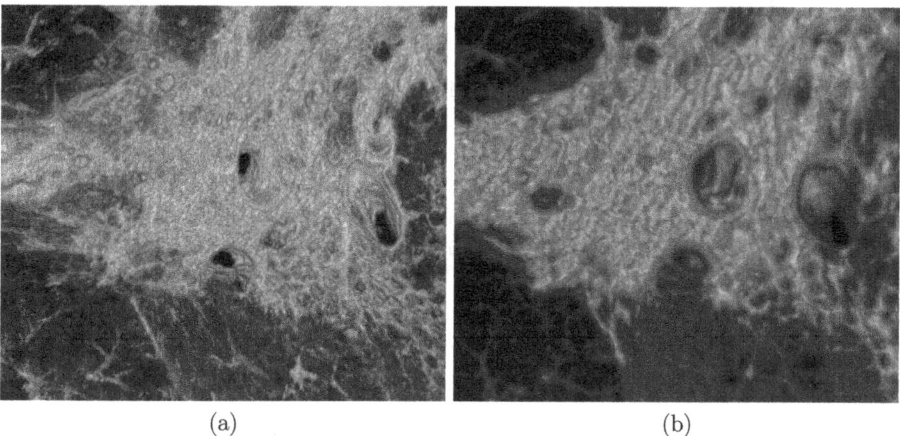

Fig. 5. Volume rendering of the reconstructed result. (a) is the histological image stack. (b) is the corresponding region in the μCT volume.

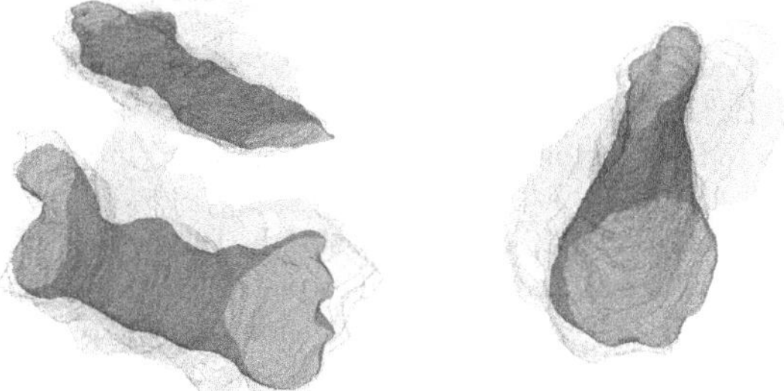

Fig. 6. Bronchial tree in the histological images and μCT volume. Red surface made from μCT volume, yellow surface extracted after initial alignment, and cyan surface extracted after non-rigid registration (Color figure online).

Table 2. Similarity comparison after alignment and non-rigid registration

		Dice Index	Jaccard Index	Recall	NCC
Case 1	Alignment	0.415	0.262	0.444	0.573
	Non-rigid	0.800	0.667	0.873	0.676
Case 2	Alignment	0.354	0.215	0.400	0.398
	Non-rigid	0.687	0.523	0.807	0.540
Mean	Alignment	0.385	0.239	0.422	0.486
	Non-rigid	0.744	0.595	0.840	0.608

4 Discussion and Conclusion

3D reconstruction from histology is difficult due to the large deformations introduced during the preparation (cutting) of the microscopic slides. In this work we proposed to first use μCT imaging before preparation of histology slides. Using the 3D information captured by μCT as guidance allows us to better recover a quality 3D reconstruction of the histological slides than when using the slides alone, as shown in our results.

The proposed reconstruction method maintains the 3D structural information by utilizing the μCT volumes. We efficiently performed global alignment by automatically skipping slices with too large deformations, followed by detailed non-rigid alignment between 2D histology slides and the 3D μCT volume.

In conclusion, a good quality 3D reconstruction of histology and its alignment with other 3D imaging modalities like μCT might ultimately facilitate the realignment with pre-operative modalities such as clinical CT and MRI imaging. We hope that this will allow us to build a bridge between microscopic and macroscopic imaging technologies. Correlating the same anatomy and pathology could allow further insight into disease progression and patient care.

Acknowledgments. Parts of this research were supported by the Kakenhi by MEXT and JSPS (26108006) and the JSPS Bilateral International Collaboration Grants.

References

1. Ceritoglu, C., Wang, L., Selemon, L.D., Csernansky, J.G., Miller, M.I., Ratnanather, J.T.: Large deformation diffeomorphic metric mapping registration of reconstructed 3D histological section images and in vivo MR images. Front. Hum. Neurosci. **4**, 43 (2010)
2. Ou, Y., Shen, D., Feldman, M., Tomaszewski, J., Davatzikos, C.: Non-rigid registration between histological and MR images of the prostate: a joint segmentation and registration framework. In: Computer Vision and Pattern Recognition Workshops, pp. 125–132. IEEE (2009)
3. Hallack, A., Papież, B.W., Wilson, J., Wang, L.M., Maughan, T., Gooding, M.J., Schnabel, J.A.: Correlating tumour histology and *ex vivo* MRI using dense modality-independent patch-based descriptors. In: Wu, G., Coupé, P., Zhan, Y., Munsell, B., Rueckert, D. (eds.) Patch-MI 2015. LNCS, vol. 9467, pp. 137–145. Springer, Cham (2015). doi:10.1007/978-3-319-28194-0_17
4. Chicherova, N., Fundana, K., Müller, B., Cattin, P.C.: Histology to μCT data matching using landmarks and a density biased RANSAC. In: Golland, P., Hata, N., Barillot, C., Hornegger, J., Howe, R. (eds.) MICCAI 2014. LNCS, vol. 8673, pp. 243–250. Springer, Cham (2014). doi:10.1007/978-3-319-10404-1_31
5. Lobachev, O., Ulrich, C., Steiniger, B.S., Wilhelmi, V., Stachniss, V., Guthe, M.: Feature-based multi-resolution registration of immunostained serial sections. Med. Image Anal. **35**, 288–302 (2017)
6. Ourselin, S., Roche, A., Subsol, G., Pennec, X., Ayache, N.: Reconstructing a 3D structure from serial histological sections. Image Vis. Comput. **19**(12), 25–31 (2001)

7. Alcantarilla, P.F., Nuevo, J., Bartoli, A.: Fast explicit diffusion for accelerated features in nonlinear scale spaces. In: British Machine Vision Conference (BMVC) (2013)
8. Glocker, B., Sotiras, A., Komodakis, N., Paragios, N.: Deformable medical image registration: setting the state of the art with discrete methods. Annu. Rev. Biomed. Eng. **13**(1), 219–244 (2011)
9. Komodakis, N., Tziritas, G., Paragios, N.: Fast, approximately optimal solutions for single and dynamic MRFs. In: Computer Vision and Pattern Recognition 2007, CVPR, pp. 1–8. IEEE (2007)
10. Rueckert, D., Sonoda, L.I., Hayes, C., Hill, D.L., Leach, M.O., Hawkes, D.J.: Non-rigid registration using free-form deformations: application to breast MR images. IEEE Trans. Med. Imaging **18**(8), 712–721 (1999)

A Neural Regression Framework for Low-Dose Coronary CT Angiography (CCTA) Denoising

Michael Green[1], Edith M. Marom[2], Nahum Kiryati[1], Eli Konen[2], and Arnaldo Mayer[2](✉)

[1] Department of Electrical Engineering, Tel-Aviv University, Tel Aviv, Israel
greenl@mail.tau.ac.il, nk@eng.tau.ac.il

[2] Diagnostic Imaging, Sheba Medical Center, Affiliated to the Sackler School of Medicine, Tel-Aviv University, Tel Aviv, Israel
{edith.marom,eli.konen, arnaldo.mayer}@sheba.health.gov.il

Abstract. In the last decade, the technological progress of multi-slice CT imaging has turned CCTA into a valuable tool for coronary assessment in many low to medium risk patients. Nevertheless, CCTA protocols expose the patient to high radiation doses, imposed by image quality and multiple cardiac phase acquisition requirements. Widespread use of CCTA calls for significant reduction of radiation exposure while maintaining high image quality as required for coronary assessment. Denoising algorithms have been recently applied to low-dose CT scans after image reconstruction. In this work, a fast neural regression framework is proposed for the denoising of low-dose CCTA. For this purpose, regression networks are trained to synthesize high-SNR patches directly from low-SNR input patches. In contrast to published methods, the denoising network is trained on real noise directly learned from noisy CT data rather than assuming a known parametric noise model. The denoised value for each pixel is computed as a function of the synthesized patches overlapping the pixel. The proposed algorithm is compared to state-of-the-art published algorithms for synthetic and real noise. The feature similarity index (FSIM) achieved by the proposed method is superior in all the comparisons with other methods, for synthetic radiation dose reductions higher than 90%. The results are further supported qualitatively, by observing a significant improvement in subsequent coronary reconstruction performed by commercial software on denoised images. The fast and high quality denoising capability suggests the proposed algorithm as a promising method for low-dose CCTA denoising.

1 Introduction

During last decade, progress in multi-slice CT imaging technology has been dramatic. The leap from 16 to 256 slices (and more) per detector has turned CCTA into a clinical reality [1]. Although it has not replaced coronary angiography, CCTA is the method of choice for many indications in low-to-medium risk patients [2]. Nevertheless, CCTA protocols expose the patient to large effective radiation doses that can reach 10 mSv [3]. Besides image quality requirements, radiation exposure is also increased by the

© Springer International Publishing AG 2017
G. Wu et al. (Eds.): Patch-MI 2017, LNCS 10530, pp. 102–110, 2017.
DOI: 10.1007/978-3-319-67434-6_12

need to acquire several scans, at different phases (multiphase acquisition) of the cardiac cycle, in order to select the phase with fewer motion artifacts [4].

Denoising of low-dose CT after image reconstruction has been investigated in several recent papers, with patch-based methods showing the most promising results [5–7]. Patch-based methods for denoising can be divided into three major approaches, depending on the source of self-similar patches used for denoising: (1) patches found in the original noisy image [5], (2) patches provided by an external model [8] or database [6], and (3) patches synthesized by a neural network [7]. In [5], the well-known BM3D algorithm was used to denoise low-dose CCTA images, performing initial noise-variance estimation using wavelet-based methods.

Using an external patch database may prove advantageous for denoising purpose as its patches may be selected to have a high SNR, not available in self-similar patches from the original noisy image. In [8], external and internal patch priors are exploited jointly. A GMM prior is learned on external clean image patches. The GMM prior is used for the clustering of noisy image patches which is followed by a low-rank approximation process for the estimation of the image recovery subspace. In [6], an external database of 2-D patches extracted from high-SNR CT scans is generated offline. For an input noisy image, all its overlapping 5×5 patches are extracted and associated, by approximate nearest-neighbors (ANN), to a high-SNR patch of the external database. Each denoised pixel is then computed as a function of the retrieved high-SNR patches that contain it.

The size of the patch database is a practical limitation even with ANN based algorithms. Recently, neural networks have been proposed for the image denoising task. In [7], a 3-layer convolutional neural network (CNN) is trained using sets of clean and noisy CT patches pairs. The noisy images are obtained by addition of Poisson noise (in the sinogram domain) to the clean images before patch extraction. Given a noisy input patch, the network is trained to generate an output patch similar to its corresponding clean patch using the L_2 distance metric. Full image denoising is obtained by feeding the trained network directly with a noisy image instead of patches.

In this work, a fast neural regression framework is proposed for the denoising of low-dose coronary CT angiography (CCTA). Regression networks are trained to synthesize high-SNR patches directly from low-SNR input patches. In contrast to published methods, the denoising network is trained on real noise directly learned from noisy CCTA, without assuming a known parametric noise model. The high SNR patches, synthesized by the regression network, are used to compute a denoised value for each CCTA pixels while preserving local structures. The remainder of this paper is organized as follows: The proposed algorithm is detailed in Sect. 2 and validated for synthetic and real noise in Sect. 3. A discussion concludes the paper in Sect. 4.

2 Methods

The proposed method (Fig. 1) is composed of two main steps: offline training of the neural framework (top) and denoising of the input low-dose CT image (bottom). Both steps will be detailed in the following subsections.

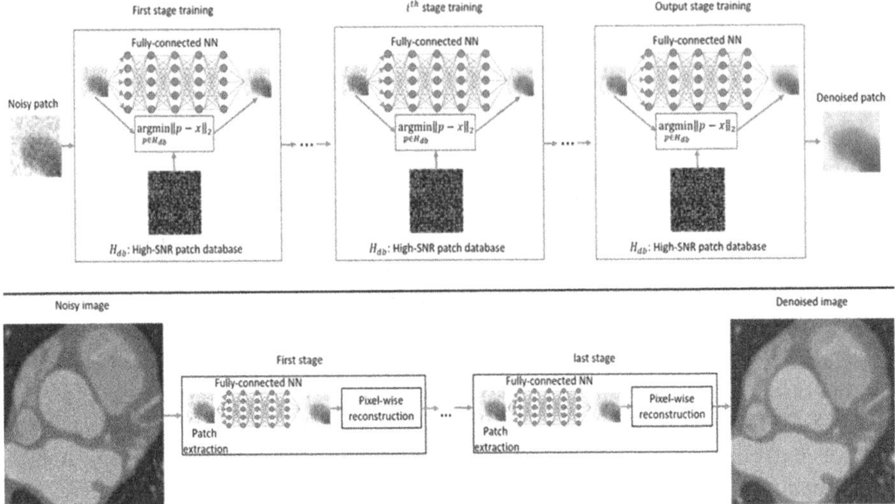

Fig. 1. The main steps of the proposed method; (top) offline training of the neural framework; (bottom) denoising of the input low-dose CT image.

2.1 Training of the Neural Framework

In the offline learning step, a neural network is trained to approximate the mapping between noisy, low-SNR patches to the clean, high-SNR patches. For this multidimensional regression task, the universal approximation property [9] of multi-layer feed-forward neural networks is particularly advantageous. Learning is performed on two groups of patches $X = \{x_i\}_{i=1}^{N}$ and $Y = \{y_i\}_{i=1}^{N}$ which denote the vectorized low-SNR patches and their corresponding high-SNR patches, respectively.

In contrast to published neural denoising methods, we propose to learn noise characteristics from real CCTA data instead of using an explicit noise model. For this purpose, instead of generating the noisy patches by artificial addition of synthetic noise to high-SNR patches, we devise the following approach: Let H_{db} and L_{db} denote two databases of high and low SNR patches, respectively. The two databases were created by random sampling of several high-SNR and low-SNR CCTA images, accordingly. We stress that the selected low-SNR images are intrinsically noisy and not the result of synthetic noise addition. The high-SNR patch, $y \in H_{db}$, corresponding to patch $x \in L_{db}$, is given by

$$y = \underset{p\in H_{db}}{\operatorname{argmin}} \|p - x\|_2 \tag{1}$$

The mapping between similar low and high-SNR CCTA patches may be efficiently implemented using an approximate nearest neighbor (ANN) algorithm.

The selected network architecture consists of 5 fully-connected layers including $n_i, i = 1..5$, neurons in each layer. Each layer performs the following computation:

$$O_i = RELU(W_i \cdot I_i + b_i) \tag{2}$$

Here W_i are the weights of layer *i*, I_i is the output of the previous layer, b_i are the biases of layer *i* and $RELU(x)$ is the commonly used activation function $\max(0, x)$. In our case, the *RELU* function is more appropriate than the *sigmoid* or *tanh* as these functions scale the output of each layer to a different range, which is undesirable for a regression task. Intuitively, the chance of finding good matches between low and high-SNR patches by ANN, decreases as patch size increases. In this *small patch* scenario, fully connected layers are preferable over convolutional ones.

The network parameters are optimized using an Euclidean cost function $C(X, Y, \theta)$:

$$C(X, Y, \theta) = \frac{1}{N}\sum_{i=1}^{N} \|F(x_i, \theta) - y_i\|_2 \tag{3}$$

Here, N is the number of training samples, θ represents the network parameters, and F is the network output. Optimization is computed by batch gradient descent. We note that no normalization of the patch values is required given the absolute character of the Hounsfield units.

In order to further enhance the denoising effect, the network described above can be cascaded into multiple denoising stages as shown in Fig. 1 (top). The networks for all the denoising stages share the same architecture, but the parameters are learned by training each denoising stage sequentially as follows: After completion of network training in the first stage, the whole noisy patches training set is fed through the network and the resulting output patches are forwarded as low-SNR training patches to the second denoising stage. Here again, the corresponding high-SNR training patches are retrieved from the high-SNR patch database H_{db}. In the proposed cascade approach, each denoising stage comprises a network specifically trained to denoise patches generated by the previous denoising stage. This is conceptually superior to iteratively denoising the patches with a single network since its training is only optimal for the first denoising iteration. The advantage will also be confirmed in the experimental results.

2.2 Denoising of Low Dose *(LD)* Scans

Given an input low-SNR CT image (Fig. 1, bottom), dense sampling of all the *SxS* patches in the image is performed. The extracted patches are then forwarded through the regression neural network to generate the corresponding high-SNR patches.

At each pixel, a denoised value is computed using the generated high-SNR patches: as shown in Fig. 2 for $S = 3$, any given pixel (grey) in the noisy image belongs simultaneously to S^2 overlapping *SxS* patches. Since a high-SNR patch was associated to each patch in the original image, a distinct high-SNR value is provided for the given pixel by each one of the S^2 overlapping patches. The denoised pixel value can then be computed as a weighted sum of these S^2 high-SNR values as suggested in [6]. Let $X_j = \{x_{j,i}\}_{i=1}^{S^2}$ denote the set of vectorized overlapping patches containing a given noisy pixel p_j, and $\hat{X}_j = F(X_j, \theta)$ be the output of the neural network for each of the patches $x_{j,i}$. The corresponding denoised value $\hat{p}_j$ can be computed by

$$\hat{p}_j = G(\hat{X}_j) = \frac{\sum_{i=1}^{S^2} \exp\left(-\frac{D(x_{j,k}, \hat{x}_{j,i})}{h^2}\right) \hat{x}_{j,i,\hat{x}}}{\sum_{i=1}^{S^2} \exp\left(-\frac{D(x_{j,k}, \hat{x}_{j,i})}{h^2}\right)} \tag{4}$$

Here, $D(P, Q)$ is the mean L_1 distance between corresponding pixels in partially overlapping patches P and Q, $k = ceil\left(\frac{S^2}{2}\right)$ is the index for the patch centered in p_j and $\hat{k}$ is the index of p_j in the vectorized patch $\hat{x}_{j,i}$. The adopted weighting scheme was chosen as it favors the preservation of local structure: the contribution of the high-SNR patches to $\hat{p}_j$ increases with their similarity to the patch centered in p_j [6].

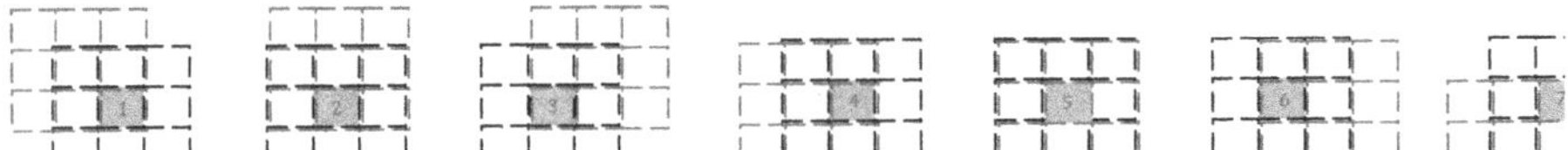

Fig. 2. A given pixel (gray) in the noisy image belongs to S^2 overlapping *SxS* patches. Here, $S = 3$. (Adapted from [6].)

The denoising steps described above constitute a denoising stage. Several denoising stages may be cascaded (Fig. 1, bottom) to enhance the overall denoising effect. At each stage, the regression network that was purposely trained (see Subsect. 2.1) is used to generate the required high-SNR patches. We stress that since a denoised image is reconstructed after each patch-denoising network (Fig. 1 bottom), the proposed cascade approach is not equivalent to training a single network that appends all the patch denoising networks defined above.

3 Experiments

For the quantitative validation of the algorithms, 40 low-dose CCTA scans (voxel size $0.29 \times 0.29 \times 0.8$ mm^3) were generated by addition of zero-mean white Gaussian noise ($\sigma = 2000$) to the sinograms of 40 real high-SNR scans. The scans, acquired under automatic exposure, were visually inspected to assess image quality. The equivalent radiation dose reduction is given by [10]:

$$R(\%) = 100 \cdot \left(1 - \frac{1}{N^2}\right) \tag{5}$$

where N is the noise ratio, approximated by a local standard deviations ratio. N is measured in a single-tissue ROI sampled in both images. In our experiments, the average dose reduction, R, computed over several single-tissue ROIs, was about 90%. The patch size S was set to 5 in all the experiments. 40 Neural networks were trained using a leave-one-out scheme. Each network was tested on a different case (out of the

40), after having been trained on a set of 10 million patches extracted from the remaining 39 cases. The numbers of neurons are set to $n_1 = 512$, $n_2 = 128$, $n_3 = 100$, $n_4 = 50$, *and* $n_5 = 25$, for the output layer, that corresponds to the size of the input 5×5 patches. Learning rate in network optimization was set to 0.0001, batch size was set to 128. Two cascaded denoising stages were used. The feature similarity index (FSIM) [11] was used for quantitative comparison between each original high-SNR image and the resulting denoised image. The FSIM index relies on ability of the human visual system to understand images from low-level features.

In Table 1, the performance of the proposed algorithm is compared for different configurations on a subset of 10 cases: synthetic/real noise in L_{db}, number of cascaded denoising stages (denoted *stg*), and number of algorithm iterations (denoted *it*). Since the two-stage configuration, trained using real noise in L_{db}, outperformed the other configurations, we will use this configuration in all the experiments and denote it NNRR2.

Table 1. Averaged *FSIM* for 10 cardiac CT scans for different configurations of our algorithm

configs	#stg = 1, #it = 1 synthetic noise	#stg = 1, #it = 2 synthetic noise	#stg = 2, #it = 2 synthetic noise	#stg = 1, #it = 1 real noise	#stg = 1, #it = 2 real noise	#stg = 2, #it = 2 real noise
Mean	0.871	0.817	0.850	0.848	0.873	**0.876**
STD	0.015	0.033	0.025	0.009	0.008	0.008

In Fig. 3, the proposed NNRR2 is compared against four state-of-the-art algorithms: BM3D [5], PGPD [8], LC-NLM [6], and CHEN [7] for the 40 scans synthetic noise database created above. Implementation codes were openly provided by the authors, except for [7], that we implemented according to the paper. The average FSIM for the proposed NNRR2 (0.87) was superior to all the compared methods. Only in 6 out of 40 cases, CHEN [7] performed equally or slightly better than NNRR2. However, it is important to note that, for fairness, CHEN was trained on the same noise model and intensity (σ) that was applied to generate the synthetic data. In practice, this

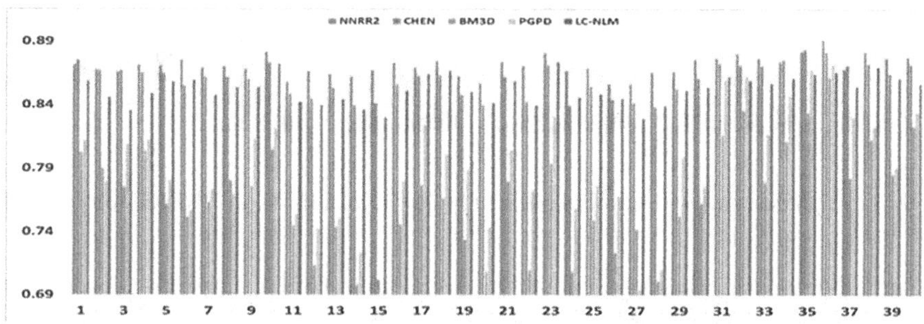

Fig. 3. The FSIM index for the 40 CCTA cases obtained with BM3D (grey), PGPD (yellow), LC-NLM (green), CHEN (orange) and NNRR2 (blue). (Color figure online)

optimal situation is infrequent. In Fig. 4, a sample slice is shown before noise addition (a), after noise addition (b), and following denoising by BM3D (c), PGPD (d), LC-NLM (e), CHEN (f), and NNRR2 (g). While BM3D (c) and PGPD (d) provide powerful denoising, the resulting images appear strongly over-smoothed when compared to the original image (a). This is best visualized in the zoomed views (g), where the capital letters associate them to the corresponding sub-image of Fig. 4. Both LC-NLM (e,E) and NNRR2 (g,G) have good visual similarity with the original image (a,A). CHEN (F) performance in the example is relatively similar to NNRR2. However, In Fig. 5, we can see how CHEN's performance (c) degrades significantly when the training noise value (σ = 2000) is not adjusted to the actual noise level (σ = 3000) in the image (b). In contrast, NNRR2 (d) still perform superior denoising independently of the actual noise level in the input image, as no assumption is made about it. The advantage is best viewed in the zoomed ROIs (e). Overall, NNRR2 demonstrates the best balance between denoising and similarity to the original image (a,A) as reflected quantitatively by the FSIM values. The average slice denoising time for NNRR2 was about 4 s in non-optimized Matlab-Python.

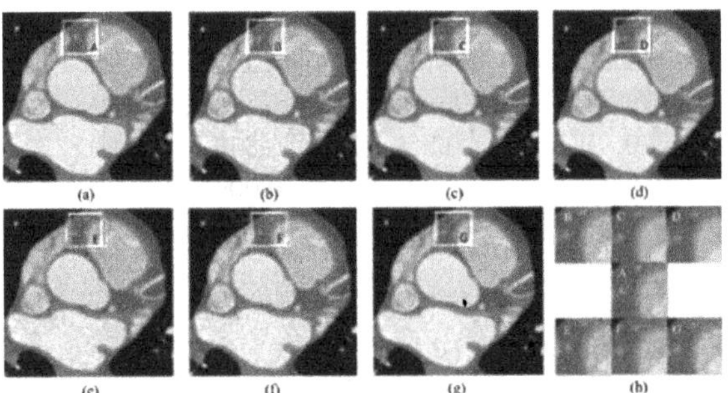

Fig. 4. A sample slice is shown before noise addition (a), after noise addition (b), and following denoising by BM3D (c), PGPD (d), LC-NLM (e), CHEN (f), and NNRR2 (g), (h) zoomed ROI: the high-SNR ROI (A) was placed in the middle for easy comparison with other ROIs (B to G).

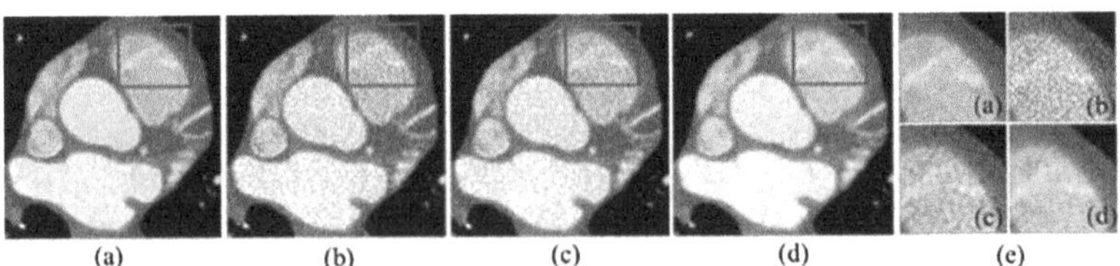

Fig. 5. (a) High dose; (b) with artificial noise (σ = 3000); (c) CHEN; (d) NNRR2; (e) Zoom-in.

To further validate the proposed method, a real noisy CCTA scan was considered in Fig. 6. The noisy scan was acquired at a phase equal to 45% of the R-R interval in the cardiac cycle. A noisy sample slice is shown (top, left) beside the corresponding 3-D reconstruction of heart and coronaries (center, right) by the Intellispace Portal cardiac

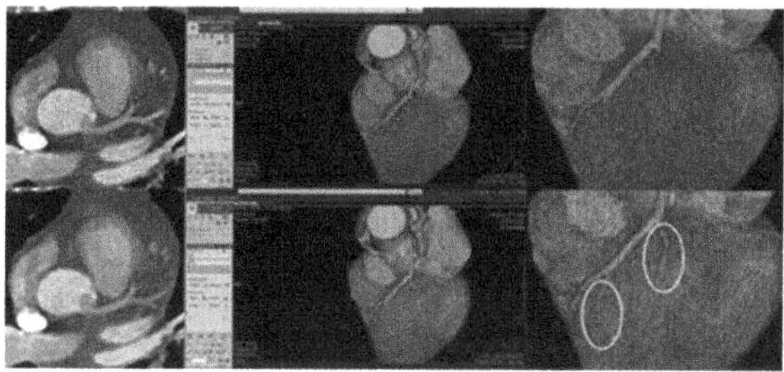

Fig. 6. (top): Real noisy sample slice (left) and 3D coronary reconstruction (center, right); (bottom) same after denoising by NNRR2. The additional coronary branches reconstructed on the denoised scan are contoured (yellow). (Color figure online)

CT software (Philips, Holland). Following denoising by NNRR2 (bottom, left) of the same scan, we observe that two additional branches of the coronaries (yellow contours) were successfully reconstructed without human intervention.

4 Conclusions

We presented a novel patch-based method for the denoising of low-dose CT, and demonstrated its applicability to the denoising of low-dose CCTA. The method relies on a fast neural regression framework that is trained to generate high-SNR patches from low-SNR input patches. The high SNR patches, synthesized by the regression network, are used to compute a denoised value for each CCTA pixel while preserving local structures in the reconstructed image. In contrast to previous methods, no assumption is made on the nature or model of the noise which is instead learned directly from real noisy data. The presented method demonstrated promising results and outperformed both quantitatively and visually other state-of-the-art algorithms in CCTA denoising, for synthetic radiation dose reductions above 90%. In ongoing research, the method will be further validated on larger datasets. Moreover, the database of low-dose patches will be enriched with real low-dose patches extracted from scans acquired at very low-dose to enhance the denoising power of the method.

References

1. Panetta, D.: Advances in X-ray detectors for clinical and preclinical computed tomography. Nucl. Instrum. Methods Phys. Res. Sect. A: Accel. Spectrom. Detect. Assoc. Equip. **809**, 2–12 (2016)
2. Stefanini, G.G., Windecker, S.: Can coronary computed tomography angiography replace invasive angiography? Circulation **131**(4), 418–426 (2015)
3. Sun, Z., Sabarudin, A.: Coronary CT angiography: state of the art. World J. Cardiol. **5**(12), 442 (2013)

4. Joemai, R.M., Geleijns, J., Veldkamp, W.J., de Roos, A., Kroft, L.J.: Automated cardiac phase selection with 64-MDCT coronary angiography. Am. J. Roentgenol. **191**(6), 1690–1697 (2008)
5. Kang, D., Slomka, P., Nakazato, R., Woo, J., Berman, D.S., Kuo, C.-C.J., Dey, D.: Image denoising of low-radiation dose coronary CT angiography by an adaptive block-matching 3D algorithm. In: SPIE Medical Imaging. International Society for Optics and Photonics (2013)
6. Green, M., Marom, E.M., Kiryati, N., Konen, E., Mayer, A.: Efficient low-dose CT denoising by locally-consistent non-local means (LC-NLM). In: Ourselin, S., Joskowicz, L., Sabuncu, M.R., Unal, G., Wells, W. (eds.) MICCAI 2016. LNCS, vol. 9902, pp. 423–431. Springer, Cham (2016). doi:10.1007/978-3-319-46726-9_49
7. Chen, H., Zhang, Y., Zhang, W., Liao, P., Li, K., Zhou, J., Wang, G.: Low-dose CT via convolutional neural network. Biomed. Opt. Express **8**(2), 679–694 (2017)
8. Chen, F., Zhang, L., Yu, H.: External patch prior guided internal clustering for image denoising. In: IEEE ICCV (2015)
9. Hornik, K., Stinchcombe, M., White, H.: Multilayer feedforward networks are universal approximators. Neural Netw. **2**(5), 359–366 (1989)
10. McNitt-Gray, M.F.: AAPM/RSNA physics tutorial for residents: topics in CT: radiation dose in CT 1. Radiographics **22**(6), 1541–1553 (2002)
11. Zhang, L., Zhang, L., Mou, X., Zhang, D.: FSIM: a feature similarity index for image quality assessment. IEEE Trans. Image Process. **20**(8), 2378–2386 (2011)

A Dictionary Learning-Based Fast Imaging Method for Ultrasound Elastography

Manyou Ma(✉), Robert Rohling, and Lutz Lampe

Department of Electrical and Computer Engineering,
The University of British Columbia, Vancouver, Canada
{manyoum,rohling,lampe}@ece.ubc.ca

Abstract. Ultrasound elastography is an imaging modality that computes the elasticity of tissue through measuring shear waves from a mechanical excitation using pulse-echo ultrasound. To better measure shear waves and reduce acquisition time, elastography would benefit from a higher framerate, which is limited by conventional focused line-by-line acquisition. This paper proposes a dictionary learning-based framework that increases the framerate of steady state elastography. The method uses patches extracted from images with higher scanline density to train a dictionary, and uses this dictionary to interpolate images with lower scanline density collected at a faster framerate. Experiments on a tissue mimicking phantom showed when the framerate is increased 8 times, the reconstructed image using the proposed method achieved a 17.6 dB Peak Signal-to-Noise Ratio. The method was also implemented on a steady state elastography system, where elasticity measurements similar to conventional methods were obtained with a shorter total acquisition time.

Keywords: Dictionary learning · Fast imaging · Ultrasound elastography

1 Introduction

Ultrasound (US) elastography, an emerging imaging modality, measures tissues' mechanical properties, such as elasticity (Young's Modulus) and viscosity, through calculating their response to external excitation forces using standard pulse-echo US. Compared to standard acoustic properties that form a B(brightness)-scan, elasticity is an adjunct at distinguishing pathology and physiological changes in tissues, such as cancer or fibrosis. There are different specific implementations of US elastography systems [10, 13]. In particular, our group previously developed a system called Shear Wave Absolute Vibro-Elastography (SWAVE) [5]. SWAVE uses an external mechanical exciter to generate harmonic vibration between 60 and 200 Hz upon the tissues (akin to magnetic resonance elastography), a US probe to collect 20 to 40 frames of pre-envelope-detected radio frequency (RF) US data at each location, and signal processing software and hardware to perform speckle tracking (or cross-correlation of RF signal

© Springer International Publishing AG 2017
G. Wu et al. (Eds.): Patch-MI 2017, LNCS 10530, pp. 111–118, 2017.
DOI: 10.1007/978-3-319-67434-6_13

windows) between subsequent frames of RF data to obtain the motion profile. The motion profile is fitted with a sinusoidal wave at the excitation frequency. From the phasor of this shear wave, inversion algorithms [6] compute the elasticity map, also called the "elastogram". Compared to Acoustic Radiation Force Impulse-based elastography methods [10], SWAVE has the advantage of using standard delay-and-sum pulse-echo beamforming, requiring no modification to US hardware, achieving deeper penetration, and providing results over the full field of view [8].

However, since there is a need to capture the fast moving tissue under fast excitations (e.g. 200 Hz) in steady state harmonic elastography, a high US framerate is required to accurately measure the motion phasor and hence the elasticity. Imaging at the framerate required for SWAVE, namely the Nyquist rate of two times the excitation frequency or higher, is impossible using conventional US machines, which currently typically have the framerate of <100 Hz. To circumvent this problem, sector-based sampling [5], which estimates the elasticity in multiple sub-sectors, and bandpass-sampling [1], which uses multiple cycles of high frequency motion to estimate the motion phasor have previously been proposed. However, both of these methods do not reduce the overall acquisition time, and the sector-based method requires multiple steps of compensation, which leads to discontinuities in the presence of cardiac and breathing motion artifacts. A more fundamental solution is to improve the inherent framerate of the US imaging system, where recent research [7,12,14] explored designing more powerful hardware, such as larger memory card and the ability to perform parallel computations, in order to conduct multiline beamforming methods. However, all of these methods are subject to increased cost required for the corresponding hardware upgrade. Given the proliferation of low-cost US systems with standard delay-and-sum beamformers, there is a need to find a solution to the speed problem with existing beamformers.

In this work, we propose a software-based approach that improves the framerate of the US system with standard beamformers and retains the ability to interleave B-mode US imaging with SWAVE scanning. To achieve this, we obtain images at a faster framerate by only taking a subset of the scanlines during SWAVE, and reconstruct images with denser scanlines using examples from the patches of training data obtained from the interleaved full-density B-mode US scans. In the computer vision community, the problem of interpolating high-resolution images from low-resolution images is generally referred to as image super-resolution (SR). We use this term although we are not attempting sub-wavelength imaging here. Previous research has explored solutions based on multi-atlas patch matching [2], dictionary learning [4], and more recently, Deep Learning [11]. Successful SR implementations have been demonstrated on the three-dimensional magnetic resonance cardiac images [4]. As a first step to speed up SWAVE using SR, we adopt a dictionary learning-based method and reconstruct the high-resolution images using sparsity-based assumptions.

2 Methods

The overview of the methods and the algorithms proposed in this paper are shown in Fig. 1. The three aspects of our algorithm, namely (a) modifications to conventional US transmission sequence, (b) patch extraction and pre-processing, and (c) the proposed patch-based dictionary learning and sparsity-based reconstruction algorithms, will be discussed in detail in this section.

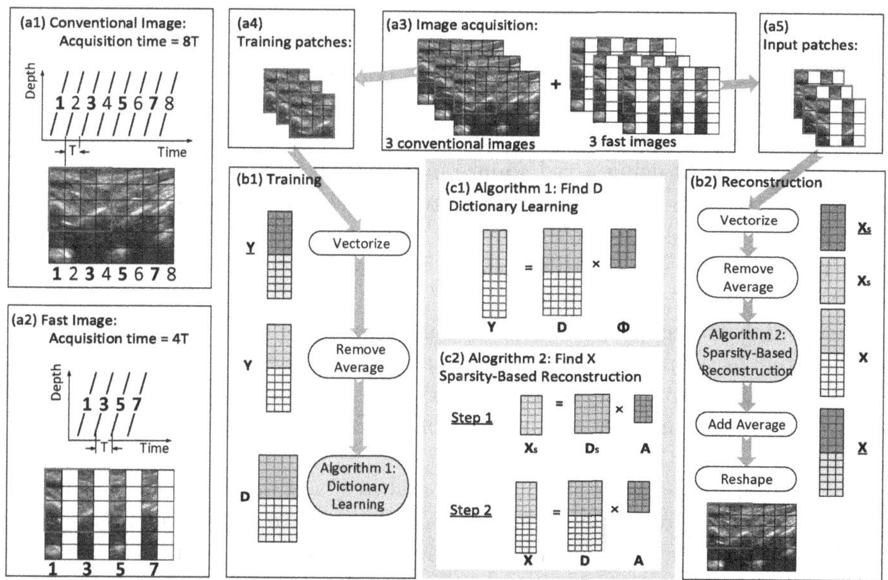

Fig. 1. Overview of the proposed methods, namely (a) modifications to conventional US transmission sequence, (b) patch extraction and pre-processing, and (c) the proposed patch-based dictionary learning and sparsity-based reconstruction algorithms. (Color figure online)

US Transmission Sequencing: Figure 1(a1) shows the conventional US transmission sequence that generates an 8-line image, where 1, 2, 3, ... 8 represent the 8 lines. The time it takes to form one of these lines depends on the speed of sound propagation in the medium and the depth of the image. Suppose it takes time T to form one line, then generating such an image takes $8T$ overall. To improve the imaging speed, in Fig. 1(a2), only every other lateral position is imaged, and the total imaging time is reduced from $8T$ to $4T$, hence a 2-fold speed-up is achieved. However, since fewer lines are acquired, the imaging lateral resolution is worse compared to the conventional images.

To improve the worsened imaging quality of the fast images, we design a learning-based approach that uses the conventional denser images as training examples to train a dictionary on-the-fly, and uses the trained dictionary to interpolate the fast images to have denser lines. To achieve this, we design a combined sequence that acquires Q conventional frames as training frames and L fast image frames subsequently. A combined sequence with $Q = 3$ and $L = 3$ is demonstrated in Fig. 1(a3). In the actual implementation, we re-arrange the transmission sequence within each conventional frame to facilitate the reconstruction step. If we denote the speed-up ratio of the fast image by P and assume that a conventional image has 128 lines, then the total acquisition time of such a sequence is $128Q \cdot T + 128L/P \cdot T$, compared to $128T \cdot L$ for the conventional US. So the overall reduction in total acquisition time is $\frac{L}{Q+L/P}$.

Overall Workflow and Pre-processing: Following methods from image SR literature [15], we use a patch-based approach to perform the learning-based interpolation. Square patches with the size $m \times m$ are extracted. A patch with $m = 4$ is highlighted using a red square in Fig. 1(a1). The extracted versions of the training patches and input patches are also demonstrated in Fig. 1(a4) and 1(a5). We re-arrange lateral lines in the training patch, so that the positions sampled by the fast images (highlighted using violet color) are put in front of the other lines.

Each patch is vectorized and the training patches and testing patches are concatenated horizontally respectively. Let us use $\underline{\boldsymbol{Y}} \in \mathbb{R}^{m^2 \times Q}$ to denote the vectorized training patches, and $\underline{\boldsymbol{X}_s} \in \mathbb{R}^{mn \times L}$ to denote the vectorized input patches, where n represents the number of lateral lines that are sampled in the fast image ($n = 2$ in Fig. 1(a4)).

The temporal average of the training patches $\underline{\boldsymbol{Y}}$ are first stored and removed, since subsequent patches are typically similar, and we are more interested in studying the minute inter-frame changes due to tissue motion. The average-removed training patches, denoted by $\boldsymbol{Y}$, are then used to train a dictionary $\boldsymbol{D} \in \mathbb{R}^{m^2 \times K}$ with K atoms, using Algorithm 1. The workflow of obtaining the dictionary from training patches is described in Fig. 1(b1), using orange arrows.

Similarly, we subtract the average of the training patches from the input patches $\underline{\boldsymbol{X}_s}$. The average removed input patches $\boldsymbol{X}_s$ are then interpolated using a subsequent sparsity-based reconstruction algorithm (Algorithm 2). We denote the output of Algorithm 2 as $\boldsymbol{X} \in \mathbb{R}^{m^2 \times L}$. After adding back the average of the training patches and re-arranging the lateral lines, patches with the same number of lateral lines as the training patches are obtained. The workflow of sparsity-based reconstruction using patches from the fast images is described in Fig. 1(b2), using green arrows.

Algorithm 1: Patch-Based Dictionary Learning: Given a series of training patches $\boldsymbol{Y} = [\boldsymbol{y}_1, \boldsymbol{y}_2, \ldots, \boldsymbol{y}_Q]$, a dictionary learning algorithm aims to find a dictionary $\boldsymbol{D} = [\boldsymbol{d}_1, \boldsymbol{d}_2, \ldots, \boldsymbol{d}_K]$, such that each training patch $\boldsymbol{y}_q$ can be represented as a linear combination with the fewest possible elements $\boldsymbol{d}_k$'s. Mathematically, this can be expressed as

$$\boldsymbol{D} = \arg\min_{\boldsymbol{D},\boldsymbol{\Phi}} \|\boldsymbol{Y} - \boldsymbol{D}\boldsymbol{\Phi}\|_2^2 + \lambda\|\boldsymbol{\Phi}\|_1, \tag{1}$$

where $\boldsymbol{\Phi} = [\boldsymbol{\phi}_1, \boldsymbol{\phi}_2, \ldots, \boldsymbol{\phi}_Q]$ and $\boldsymbol{\phi}_q \in \mathbb{R}^K$ represent the sparse code for training patch q. The dictionary learning algorithm is shown in Fig. 1(c1). There are many efficient implementations of dictionary learning algorithms in the literature. In this paper, we picked a computationally efficient toolbox [9].

Algorithm 2: Sparsity-Based Reconstruction: Our proposed sparsity-based reconstruction algorithm takes a patch $\boldsymbol{x}_{sl} \in \mathbb{R}^{mn}$ from a fast image as input, and reconstructs the higher resolution patch $\boldsymbol{x}_l \in \mathbb{R}^{m^2}$. Two constraints we use are: (1) the recovered $\boldsymbol{x}_l$ has a sparse representation $\boldsymbol{a}_l$ using dictionary $\boldsymbol{D}$; (2) the first mn elements of $\boldsymbol{x}_l$, which correspond to the sampled positions in the fast image, are similar to $\boldsymbol{x}_{sl}$. If we denote the first mn rows of $\boldsymbol{D}$ as $\boldsymbol{D}_s$, these two constraints can be expressed mathematically as

$$\begin{aligned} \underset{\boldsymbol{a}_l}{\text{minimize}} \quad & \|\boldsymbol{a}_l\|_1 \\ \text{subject to} \quad & \|\boldsymbol{D}_s \cdot \boldsymbol{a}_l - \boldsymbol{x}_{sl}\|_2^2 \leq \sigma^2, \end{aligned} \tag{2}$$

which is a Basis Pursuit Denoising setup, with σ representing the margin of error allowed, and can be solved efficiently by many compressed sensing solvers, such as SPGL-1 [3]. After the sparse codes corresponding to all the fast imaging patches are found, the reconstructed patches can be found by $\boldsymbol{X} = \boldsymbol{D}\boldsymbol{A}$, where $\boldsymbol{A} = [\boldsymbol{a}_1, \boldsymbol{a}_2, \ldots, \boldsymbol{a}_l]$. This procedure is illustrated in Fig. 1(c2).

3 Experiments

In this section, we introduce two experiments we designed to test the accuracy of the proposed combination of dictionary-learning and reconstruction methods and their applicability to SWAVE. For both experiments, we used a SonixTouch (Analogic Corp., Richmond, CA) machine and a custom made mechanical exciter. The phantom being imaged was a standard CIRS (Norfolk, VA) elasticity phantom. In-house motor control box and sequencers were used for 3D sweep imaging and accurate line-triggering.

For the first experiment, the mechanical excitation frequency was set to 200 Hz and the US framerate was set to 72 Hz. First we measured the error caused by noise and triggering error: Since for an excitation frequency f_{e} and US framerate f_{frame}, a finite set of phase locations

$$k = \frac{\mathrm{lcm}(f_{\mathrm{e}}, f_{\mathrm{frame}})}{f_{\mathrm{e}}}, \tag{3}$$

were sampled by the US machine, where lcm stands for the least common multiple, we may find that only 9 distinct locations of the excitation phases are sampled using this combination. Therefore, the frames collected should be identical every 10 frames, in the absence of measurement noise and inaccuracy of triggering. We recorded the average Peak Signal-to-Noise Ratio (PSNR) between pairs of frames that are 10 frames apart. This PSNR is measured as 13.9 dB, and will be referred to as "Error Due to Noise" and provides a bronze standard for evaluating our methods' performance. We inject a half-frame time delay before taking the fast frames, to ensure the training frames and input frames measure different phases of the motion. For each experimental setting, we collected 23 frames before injecting the delay and 4 frames after injecting the delay.

For the second experiment, we implemented the proposed method to achieve a faster SWAVE system. 15 frames of a 128-line transmission sequence were used as training images and 40 frames of a 16-line transmission sequence were used as fast images. Hence, a speed-up ratio of 8 was achieved. The total image acquisition time decreases from $40 \cdot 128T$ to $(15 + 40/8) \cdot 128T = 20 \cdot 128T$, i.e., an overall reduction in imaging time of 50% was achieved. The elastograms were derived using Local Frequency Estimation [6].

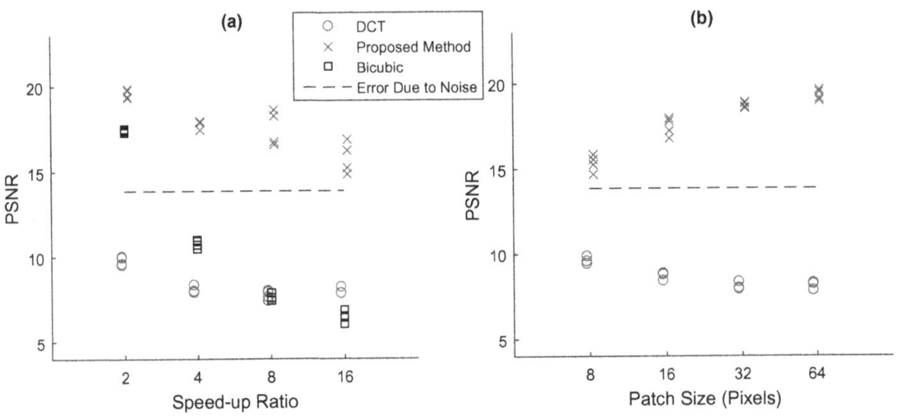

Fig. 2. (a) Reconstruction accuracy using the DCT, Bicubic interpolation, and our proposed method at different speed-up ratios. (b) Reconstruction accuracy using the DCT and our proposed method at using different patch sizes. The "Error Due to Noise" measurement is denoted by the dashed line.

In Fig. 2(a), we compare the reconstruction accuracy using our proposed dictionary learning algorithm with that using a Discrete Cosine Transform (DCT) and a Bicubic interpolation. We plot the reconstruction PSNR at different acceleration speed, compared to the previously reported "Error Due to Noise" measurement. The reconstructions using the proposed method are more accurate compared to the "Error Due to Noise" measurement. At the speed-up ratio at 2, 4, and 8, our reconstruction method out-performs the DCT and Bicubic interpolation approach. We observe that the reconstruction accuracy stays reasonable as the speed-up ratio is increased to up to 16 times. Apart from the speed-up ratio, the reconstruction accuracy is also dependent on the patch size chosen for reconstruction. In Fig. 2(b), we compare the reconstruction PSNR using patch sizes 8, 16, 32, and 64. We observe that the proposed algorithm out-performs the interpolation and DCT-based methods. In Fig. 3, we compare the elasticity measurement results obtained using the original system and the proposed fast

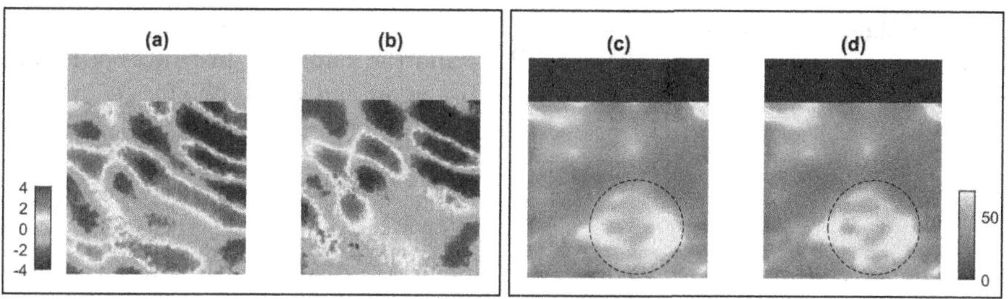

Fig. 3. (a)(c) Phasor diagram [μm] and elastogram [kPa] obtained using the conventional approach at the framerate of 72 Hz. (b)(d) Phasor diagram and elastogram obtained using the proposed method at a framerate of 576 Hz. The hard inclusion is enclosed using a dashed circle.

imaging method. The elasticity phantom has a circular hard inclusion within the field of view, which is delineated using a dashed circle. Figure 3(a) and (b) display the motion phasors gathered using the conventional method and the proposed method. We observed that good quality phasors were derived in both cases. Figure 3(c) and (d) display the elastograms gathered using the two methods. We observe similar elastograms in both cases, with a circular hard inclusion in the field of view (60.2±5.8 kPa for conventional imaging and 62.4±5.3 kPa for our proposed fast imaging method). Hence, the reconstruction PSNR achieved by the proposed method is accurate enough for elasticity measurements.

4 Discussion and Conclusion

In this paper, we proposed a fast US imaging method based on patch-based dictionary learning and sparsity-based reconstruction. In particular, this method can be used to increase the imaging speed of steady state elastography systems. We performed phantom studies and proved that when the framerate is increased 8 times, the reconstructed image using the proposed method achieved a 17.6 dB PSNR, which is higher than the 13.9 dB PSNR between two frames imaging an identical scene. We also implemented the algorithm on SWAVE, and proved that the reconstruction is accurate enough for elasticity measurements.

Our proposed method has the potential to benefit SWAVE, or other steady state elastography methods such as [13], in two aspects, the improvement in temporal sampling frequency and the reduction in total acquisition time. To test the clinical improvement in performance due to the improvement of temporal sampling rate, we will design experiments that measure elastograms of real tissue *in vivo*. Currently, in a liver elasticity exam, using a steady state elastography system, hundreds of US frames are required to generate one elastogram, during which the patient is required to perform a breath hold to avoid motion artifact. From implementing our method onto the SWAVE system, we proved that the proposed method can reduce the total acquisition time of an elastography exam, hence can reduce the potential of error from body motions.

Acknowledgement. This work was supported by the Natural Sciences and Engineering Research Council of Canada (NSERC) and the Canadian Institutes of Health Research (CIHR). We thank Drs. Mohammad Honarvar and Julio Lobo for engineering help with SWAVE.

References

1. Baghani, A., Brant, A., Salcudean, S., Rohling, R.: A high-frame-rate ultrasound system for the study of tissue motions. IEEE Trans. UFFC **57**(7), 1535–1547 (2010)
2. Bai, W., Shi, W., O'Regan, D.P., Tong, T., Wang, H., Jamil-Copley, S., Peters, N.S., Rueckert, D.: A probabilistic patch-based label fusion model for multi-atlas segmentation with registration refinement: application to cardiac MR images. IEEE Trans. Med. Imaging **32**(7), 1302–1315 (2013)
3. van den Berg, E., Friedlander, M.P.: Probing the pareto frontier for basis pursuit solutions. SIAM J. Sci. Comput. **31**(2), 890–912 (2008)
4. Bhatia, K.K., Price, A.N., Shi, W., Hajnal, J.V., Rueckert, D.: Super-resolution reconstruction of cardiac MRI using coupled dictionary learning. In: 2014 IEEE ISBI, pp. 947–950, April 2014
5. Eskandari, H., Goksel, O., Salcudean, S.E., Rohling, R.: Bandpass sampling of high-frequency tissue motion. IEEE Trans. UFFC **58**(7), 1332–1343 (2011)
6. Honarvar, M., Sahebjavaher, R.S., Rohling, R., Salcudean, S.E.: A comparison of finite element-based inversion algorithms, local frequency estimation, and direct inversion approach used in MRE. IEEE Trans. Med. Imaging **36**(8), 1686–1698 (2017). doi:10.1109/TMI.2017.2686388. ISSN 0278-0062
7. Jensen, J.A., Nikolov, S.I., Gammelmark, K.L., Pedersen, M.H.: Synthetic aperture ultrasound imaging. Ultrasonics **44**, e5–e15 (2006)
8. Lobo, J., Baghani, A., Eskandari, H., Mahdavi, S., Rohling, R., Goldernberg, L., Morris, W.J., Salcudean, S.: Prostate vibro-elastography: multi-frequency 1D over 3D steady-state shear wave imaging for quantitative elastic modulus measurement. In: 2015 IEEE IUS, pp. 1–4. IEEE (2015)
9. Mairal, J., Bach, F., Ponce, J., Sapiro, G.: Online dictionary learning for sparse coding. In: Proceedings of the 26th Annual International Conference on Machine Learning, pp. 689–696. ACM (2009)
10. Nightingale, K., Soo, M.S., Nightingale, R., Trahey, G.: Acoustic radiation force impulse imaging: in vivo demonstration of clinical feasibility. Ultrasound Med. Biol. **28**(2), 227–235 (2002)
11. Oktay, O., et al.: Multi-input cardiac image super-resolution using convolutional neural networks. In: Ourselin, S., Joskowicz, L., Sabuncu, M.R., Unal, G., Wells, W. (eds.) MICCAI 2016. LNCS, vol. 9902, pp. 246–254. Springer, Cham (2016). doi:10.1007/978-3-319-46726-9_29
12. Rabinovich, A., Friedman, Z., Feuer, A.: Multi-line acquisition with minimum variance beamforming in medical ultrasound imaging. IEEE Trans. UFFC **60**(12), 2521–2531 (2013)
13. Sinkus, R., Bercoff, J., Tanter, M., Gennisson, J.L., El Khoury, C., Servois, V., Tardivon, A., Fink, M.: Nonlinear viscoelastic properties of tissue assessed by ultrasound. IEEE Trans. UFFC **53**, 2009–2018 (2006)
14. Tanter, M., Fink, M.: Ultrafast imaging in biomedical ultrasound. IEEE Trans. UFFC **61**(1), 102–119 (2014)
15. Yang, J., Wright, J., Huang, T.S., Ma, Y.: Image super-resolution via sparse representation. IEEE Trans. Imag. Proc. **19**(11), 2861–2873 (2010)

Tumor, Lesion

Breast Tumor Detection in Ultrasound Images Using Deep Learning

Zhantao Cao[1(✉)], Lixin Duan[1], Guowu Yang[1], Ting Yue[2], Qin Chen[3], Huazhu Fu[4], and Yanwu Xu[5]

[1] The Big Data Research Center, University of Electronic Science and Technology of China, Chengdu, China
caozhantao@163.com
[2] School of Medicine, University of Electronic Science and Technology of China, Chengdu, China
[3] Sichuan Academy of Medical Sciences and Sichuan Provincial People's Hospital, University of Electronic Science and Technology of China, Chengdu, China
[4] Agency for Science, Technology and Research, Singapore, Singapore
[5] Guangzhou Shiyuan Electronics Co., Ltd., Guangzhou, China

Abstract. Detecting tumor regions in breast ultrasound images has always been an interesting topic. Due to the complex structure of breasts and the existence of noise in the ultrasound images, traditional handcraft feature based methods usually cannot achieve satisfactory results. With the recent advance of deep learning, the performance of object detection has been boosted to a great extent, especially for general object detection. In this paper, we aim to systematically evaluate the performance of several existing state-of-the-art object detection methods for breast tumor detection. To achieve that, we have collected a new dataset consisting of 579 benign and 464 malignant lesion cases with the corresponding ultrasound images manually annotated by experienced clinicians. Comprehensive experimental results clearly show that the recently proposed convolutional neural network based method, Single Shot MultiBox Detector (SSD), outperforms other methods in terms of both precision and recall.

Keywords: Deep learning · Breast tumor detection

1 Introduction

Breast cancer is the second leading cause of female death. Early diagnosis is the key for breast cancer control, as it can reduce mortality dramatically (40% or more) [1]. Previously, mammography is the main modality for detecting of breast cancer. However, mammography not only causes health risks for patients, but also leads to unnecessary (65–85%) biopsy operation due to low specificity [1]. As a much better option, ultrasound imaging can increase the overall cancer detection by 17% and reduce unnecessary biopsies by 40% [1]. Currently, using

© Springer International Publishing AG 2017
G. Wu et al. (Eds.): Patch-MI 2017, LNCS 10530, pp. 121–128, 2017.
DOI: 10.1007/978-3-319-67434-6_14

ultrasound techniques for tumor detection relies on doctor's experience, especially for the marks and measurements of tumors. Specifically, a doctor usually uses ultrasound instruments for tumor detection by first finding a good angle to wake the tumor clearly shown on the screen, and then keeping probe fixed for a long time using one hand, with another hand to mark and measure the tumor on the screen. It is a difficult task, because the slight shaking of hand holding the probe will cause big impact on the quality of breast ultrasound images; Based on this, computer aided automatic detection technology is highly demanded for locating regions of interest (ROIs), i.e., tumors, in breast ultrasound images.

Several previous methods discussed on how to automatically locate ROIs of breast tumors. In [2], A self-organizing map neural network was used for the detection of the breast tumor. The ROIs can be extracted automatically by employing local textures and a local gray level co-occurrence matrix which is a joint probability density function of two positions. Compared with the basic texture feature, the gray level co-occurrence matrix can reflect the comprehensive information about the direction, the interval and the amplitude of the image. In [3], Shan et al. developed an automatic ROI generation method which consisted of two parts: automatic seed point selection and region growing. However, the method depends on textural features, and these features are not effective for breast ultrasound images when there exists a fat region close to the tumor area or contrast is low [4]. In [5], a supervises learning method was proposed to categorize breast tissues into different classes by using a trained texture classifier, where background knowledge rules were used to select the final ROIs for the tissues. However, due to the inflexibility of the introduced constraints in the proposed method, its robustness was reduced. In [4], the authors improved the method in [5] by proposing a fully automatic and adaptive ROI generation method with flexible constraints. In their work, the ROI seed can be generated with high accuracy, and can also well distinguish the dataset tumor regions from normal regions. However, as shown in the experiments, the recall is still unsatisfactory, that average recall rate was low that benign was 27.69%, malignant was 30.91%, total was 29.29%.

Recently, deep learning techniques have attracted a lot of attention from researchers, because of the good data interpretability as well as the high discriminability power. Noticeably, deep convolutional neural networks (CNNs) have substantially improved the performance not only for image classification, but also for general object detection [6–9]. In order to take advantage of the recent developement of CNNs, in this work we employ the state-of-the-art CNN based detection methods to locate tumor regions in breast ultrasound images, and systematically evaluate them on our newly collected dataset consisting of both benign and malignant breast tumor images. So far in the literature, people have employed CNN based methods to handle detection tasks for other image modalities, such as mammograms [10]. To the best of our knowledge, there is little work that has comprehensively evaluated the performance of different CNN based detection methods for detecting tumors in breast ultrasound images. To this end, in this work we establish benchmarks for our newly collected dataset, and our study can potentially benefit other researchers working in the same area.

2 Related Work

2.1 Traditional Object Detection

The traditional object detection framework normally consists of three parts: (1) feature extraction; (2) proposal regions generation (including sliding window [11], Selective Search [12] and Objectness [13]); (3) proposal classification.

In the past, researchers usually studied hand-crafted features within the traditional detection framework. For example, Dalalet and Triggs [14] used SVM with histogram of oriented gradients (HOG) features for the pedestrian detection task. Felzenszwalb et al. [15] proposed a Deformable Part-based Model (DPM) using latent SVM, which achieved the best performance in the 2006 PASCAL person detection challenge. In [16], the authors used the K-SVD dictionary learning method to obtain a sparse expression of an image, which was called Histograms of Sparse Codes (HSC). HSC was used to replace HOG for classifier training and target detection. Although the performance has been considerably improved, the detection speed is quite slow. In [17], the author proposed an object detector based on co-occurrence features, which was three kinds of local co-occurrence features constructed by the traditional Haar, LBP, and HOG respectively. In addition, the author proposed a generalization and efficiency balanced framework for boosting training, where both high accuracy and good efficiency were achieved. Although the traditional detection method developed for many years, in recent years, it is generally acknowledged that progress has been slow.

2.2 CNN Based Object Detection

The remarkable progress of deep learning techniques, especially CNN, have largely promoted the research of visual object detection. In the following, we briefly review some state-of-the-art CNN based detection methods.

In 2014, Girshick et al. [18] proposed Region-based Convolutional Neural Networks (R-CNN), which combined the heuristic region proposal method and CNN. However, R-CNN has notable drawbacks: (1) the training phase is time-consuming; and (2) the detection phase is slow due to the repetitive feature extraction. In order to improve the speed of R-CNN, He et al. [19] introduced Spatial Pyramid Pooling Net (SPP-Net). Compared to R-CNN, SPP-Net does not require to resize proposed regions to a fixed size. Since the convolution process is done only once by caching the values, SPP-Net largely accelerates the detection time. However, two major issues still exist: (1) the training phase is quite complex; and (2) the fine-tuning stage could not update the convolutional layers, which somehow restricts SPP-Net to achieve better performance. To overcome those drawbacks, also inspired by SPP-net [19], Girshick [6] improved R-CNN by proposing Fast R-CNN which adds a ROI pooling layer to the last convolution layer as well as performs classification and bounding box regression simultaneously. However, as selective search is used for region proposals, the detection time is not very fast. To avoid the standalone step to generate regions, Ren et al. [7] proposed to integrate a so-called Region Proposal Network (RPN) into Fast R-CNN. Since the convolutional features of regions are shared, the region proposal step is almost cost free, making the detection phase of Faster R-CNN almost real-time. But the small scale objects cannot be well detected, due to the loss of detail information in the corresponding deep features.

Recently, researchers also investigated possible ways to avoid proposing regions at the very beginning for detection. For instance, You Only Look Once (YOLO) [8] employed a single convolutional neural network to predict the bounding boxes and class labels of detected regions. Since the YOLO limits the number of bounding boxes, it avoids repetitive detection of the same object and thus greatly improves the detection speed, making YOLO suitable for real-world applications. However, like Faster R-CNN, YOLO also has problems in detecting small scale objects. To deal with the issues as in YOLO, Liu et al. [9] proposed Single Shot MultiBox Detector (SSD) by generating bounding boxes of multiple sizes and aspect ratios from feature maps of different levels. However, these CNN-based methods only focus on general object detection. In this paper, we apply them to detecting tumors in our newly collected breast ultrasound dataset.

3 Dataset

Collecting a well defined dataset for breast ultrasound images is key to the research on breast tumor detection/classification. For that, we have been collaborating with Sichuan Provincial People's Hospital to have experienced clinicians annotate breast ultrasound images obtained from breast lesions patients. Specifically, the patients were told to get scanned by LOGIQ E9 (GE) and IU-Elite (PHILIPS) to generate those ultrasound images. Each ultrasound image was later reviewed and diagnosed by two or three clinicians. Based on the ratings obtained from the BI-RADS system [22], each diagnosed image was then grouped into 7 categories indexed from 0 to 6, where 0 means more information is needed, 1 negative, 2 benign finding, 3 probably benign (less than 2% likelihood of cancer), 4 suspicious abnormality, 5 highly suggestive of malignancy, and 6 proven malignancy. According to [22], some medical specialists proposed to further partition the fourth category (suspicious abnormality) into three sub-category, i.e., 4A (low suspicion for malignancy), 4B (intermediate suspicion of malignancy) and 4C (moderate concern, but not obvious for malignancy). For that, by following the professional instructions from our clinicians, we divide our dataset into two classes: benign and malignant. The benign class is constructed by the images grouped into categories 2, 3 and 4A, while the malignant class consists of the images from categories 4B, 4C, 5 and 6.

By working with the clinicians, we have collected 579 benign and 464 malignant cases from patients. Moreover, the tumor in each image has also been marked out by those experienced clinicians. Figure 1 showcases four ultrasound

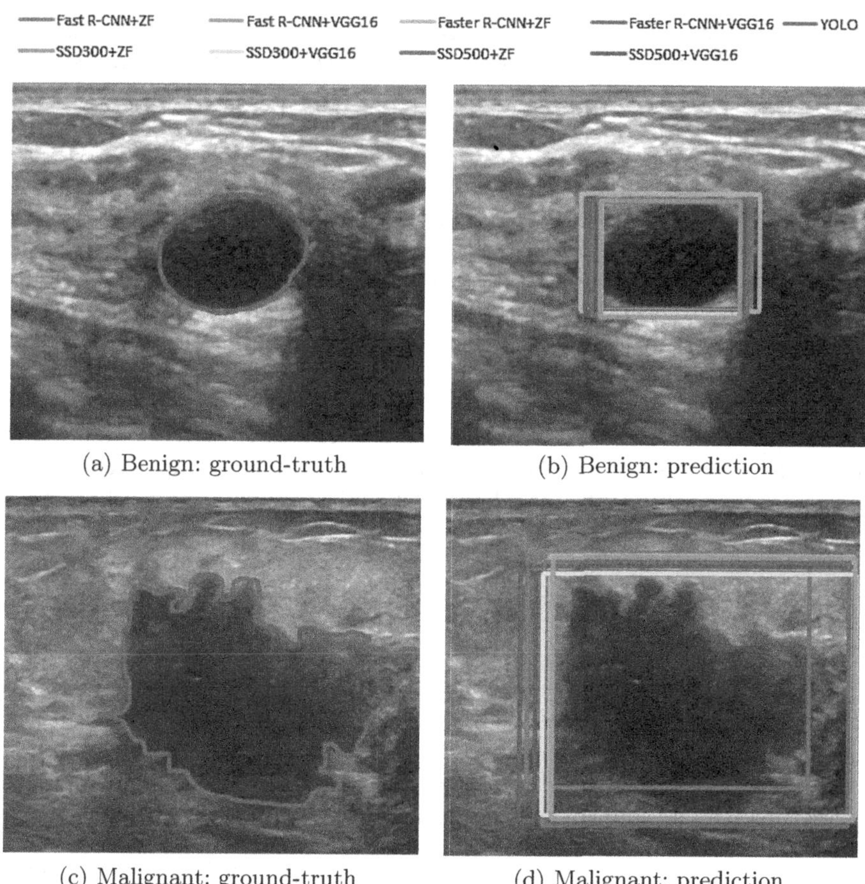

Fig. 1. Ground-truth annotations and predicted bounding boxes of different methods, for four tumor cases from different patients.

images containing either benign or malignant tumors. To the best of our knowledge, there is no such a publicly available ultrasound image dataset as ours for breast tumors.

4 Experiments

4.1 Experimental Setup

In the experiments, we evaluate the performance of several state-of-the-art detection methods, i.e., Fast R-CNN [6], Faster R-CNN [7], YOLO [8], and SSD [9]. We also combine each CNN based detection method with different existing neural networks, e.g., VGG16 [20], ZFNet [21].

For evaluation metric, we employ average precision rate (APR) and average recall rate (ARR) over all test images [4] as well as the F_1 score for each method:

$$\mathrm{APR} = \frac{1}{N}\sum_{i=1}^{N}\frac{\left|R_i^{gt} \cap R_i^{pred}\right|}{\left|R_i^{pred}\right|}, \quad \mathrm{ARR} = \frac{1}{N}\sum_{i=1}^{N}\frac{\left|R_i^{gt} \cap R_i^{pred}\right|}{\left|R_i^{gt}\right|}, \quad \mathrm{F}_1 = \frac{2 \times \mathrm{APR} \times \mathrm{ARR}}{\mathrm{APR} + \mathrm{ARR}},$$

where N is the number of images, R_i^{gt} is the grount-truth tumor region, and R_i^{pred} is the predicted bounding box. A higher APR shows the higher overlapped rate between the ROI and the true tumor region, while a higher ARR indicates that ROI generated by the proposed method could be subject to the removal of additional non-tumor regions.

In the experiments, we prepare our data as follows. For the benign class, 285 cases are randomly selected as the training set, 191 cases as the validation set and 103 cases as the test set. For the malignant class, we sample 230 cases as training set, 154 cases as the validation set and 80 cases as test set. In total, we have 515 training cases, 345 validation cases and 183 test cases. It's worth noting that all experimental protocols were approved by Sichuan Academy of Medical Sciences and Sichuan Provincial People's Hospital.

4.2 Results

In this paper, we compared the results of the different methods (the method in [4], Fast R-CNN, Faster R-CNN, YOLO, SSD) on the locating tumor ROIs in breast ultrasound images. For the deep architecture, we employ a medium-sized network VGG16 [20] and a small network ZFNet [21] for Fast R-CNN, Faster R-CNN and SSD. YOLO uses its original Darknet model [8].

The comparison of these baseline is listed in Table 1, where the APRs, ARRs and F_1 scores of different methods are compared on three settings, i.e., benign

Table 1. Average precision rates (APR), average recall rates (ARR) and F_1 scores of different methods under three settings.

Method	Benign			Malignant			Benign + Malignant		
	APR	ARR	F_1	APR	ARR	F_1	APR	ARR	F_1
Fully auto ROI [4]	66.95	14.16	23.38	78.22	19.23	30.87	71.86	16.36	26.65
Fast R-CNN+ZFNet	87.25	65.47	74.81	89.02	53.54	66.86	91.11	62.60	74.21
Fast R-CNN+VGG16	90.17	66.39	76.47	71.00	40.83	51.84	88.70	61.97	72.96
Faster R-CNN+ZFNet	93.14	66.25	77.43	86.37	46.83	60.73	92.42	62.23	74.38
Faster R-CNN+VGG16	93.01	67.08	77.95	90.36	52.05	66.05	92.37	62.54	74.58
YOLO	95.59	68.85	80.05	96.46	57.73	72.23	96.81	65.83	78.37
SSD300+ZFNet	**97.20**	**70.56**	**81.76**	96.44	54.91	69.97	**96.89**	**67.23**	**79.38**
SSD300+VGG16	96.03	69.76	80.82	**97.56**	**58.96**	**73.50**	96.42	66.70	78.85
SSD500+ZFNet	95.98	70.04	80.98	94.22	54.90	69.38	95.09	65.06	77.26
SSD500+VGG16	94.58	69.57	80.17	94.67	55.82	70.23	96.42	66.70	78.85

images only, malignant images only and both benign + malignant images. We can clearly observe that the CNN based methods perform much better than the method in [4]. Also, SSD300 in general achieves good results than other CNN based methods, which shows SSD300 is more suitable for the tumor detection task in this work. It is worth noting that SSD300 is better than SSD500 in all three settings by using either ZFNet or VGG16. The reason is as follows. SSD300 resizes images into 300×300, while SSD500 makes the size as 500×500. The region candidates in SSD300 cover a relatively larger area than those in SSD500. Since the tumor region takes a good portion in an image, SSD300 is able to better capture the region, which thus leads to better performance. Furthermore, SSD300+ZFNet is better than SSD300+VGG16 under the benign setting, but worse under the malignant setting. This interesting observation can be explained based on the model complexity of ZFNet and VGG16. Specifically, although ZFNet is a small neural network, it can well handle the easier case (i.e., benign), but is a bit underfitting for the harder case (i.e., malignant). In contrast, the larger VGG16 model is good at dealing with malignant tumors, while getting overfitting for the benign ones.

We also plot the resultant bounding boxes predicted by different methods for four tumor cases in Fig. 1.

5 Conclusion and Future Work

In this paper, we have mainly studied the existing state-of-the-art CNN based methods for tumor detection in breast ultrasound images. Due to the lack of publicly available dataset, we have collected a new one consisting of both benign and malignant cases, which are carefully annotated by experienced clinicians. Through comprehensive experiments, we find that SSD300 achieves the best performance in terms of APR, ARR and F_1 score.

Currently in our work, we only detected the tumor regions by using bounding boxes. In the future, we will conduct further investigation on the automatic segmentation of tumor areas.

Acknowledgement. This work is supported by grants from the National Natural Science Foundation of China (61572109) and the Fundamental Research Funds for the Central Universities (ZYGX2016J164).

References

1. Cheng, H.D., Shan, J., Ju, W., Guo, Y.H., Zhang, L.: Automated breast cancer detection and classification using ultrasound images: a survey. Pattern Recogn. **43**, 299–317 (2010)
2. Su, Y., Wang, Y.: Automatic detection of the region of interest from breast tumor ultrasound image. Chin. J. Biomed. Eng. **29**(2), 178–184 (2010)
3. Shan, J., Cheng, H.D., Wang, X.Y.: Completely automated segmentation approach for breast ultrasound images using multiple-domain features. Ultrasound Med. Biol. **38**(2), 262–275 (2012)

4. Xian, M., Zhang, Y.T., Cheng, H.D.: Fully automatic segmentation of breast ultrasound images based on breast characteristics in space and frequency domains. Pattern Recogn. **48**(2), 485–497 (2015)
5. Liu, B., Cheng, H.D., Huang, J.H., Tian, J.W., Tang, X.L., Liu, J.F.: Fully automatic and segmentation-robust classification of breast tumors based on local texture analysis of ultrasound images. Pattern Recogn. **43**(1), 280–298 (2010)
6. Girshick, R.: Fast R-CNN. In: ICCV, pp. 1440–1448 (2015)
7. Ren, S.Q., He, K., Girshick, R., Sun, J.: Faster R-CNN: towards real-time object detection with region proposal networks. In: NIPS (2015)
8. Redmon, J., Divvala, S.K., Girshick, R., Farhadi, A.: You only look once: unified, real-time object detection. In: CVPR, pp. 779–788 (2015)
9. Liu, W., Anguelov, D., Erhan, D., Szegedy, C., Reed, S., Fu, C.-Y., Berg, A.C.: SSD: single shot MultiBox detector. In: Leibe, B., Matas, J., Sebe, N., Welling, M. (eds.) ECCV 2016. LNCS, vol. 9905, pp. 21–37. Springer, Cham (2016). doi:10.1007/978-3-319-46448-0_2
10. Akselrod-Ballin, A., Karlinsky, L., Alpert, S., Hasoul, S., Ben-Ari, R., Barkan, E.: A region based convolutional network for tumor detection and classification in breast mammography. In: Carneiro, G., et al. (eds.) LABELS/DLMIA -2016. LNCS, vol. 10008, pp. 197–205. Springer, Cham (2016). doi:10.1007/978-3-319-46976-8_21
11. Viola, P., Jones, M.: Robust real-time face detection. In: IJCV (2004)
12. Sande, K., Uijlings, J., Gevers, T., Smeulders, A.: Segmentation as selective search for object recognition. In: ICCV (2011)
13. Alexe, B., Deselaers, T., Ferrari, V.: What is an object? In: CVPR (2010)
14. Dalal, N., Triggs, B.: Histograms of oriented gradients for human detection. In: CVPR (2005)
15. Felzenszwalb, P., McAllester, D., Ramaman, D.: A discriminatively trained and multiscale: deformable part model. In: CVPR, pp. 1–8 (2008)
16. Ren, X.F., Ramanan, D.: Histograms of sparse codes for object detection. In: CVPR, pp. 3246–3253 (2013)
17. Ren, H.Y., Li, Z.N.: Object detection using generalization and efficiency balanced co-occurrence features. In: ICCV, pp. 46–54 (2015)
18. Girshick, R., Donahue, J., Darrell, T., Malik, J.: Rich feature hierarchies for accurate object detection and semantic segmentation. In: CVPR, pp. 580–587 (2014)
19. He, K., Zhang, X., Ren, S., Sun, J.: Spatial pyramid pooling in deep convolutional networks for visual recognition. In: Fleet, D., Pajdla, T., Schiele, B., Tuytelaars, T. (eds.) ECCV 2014. LNCS, vol. 8691, pp. 346–361. Springer, Cham (2014). doi:10.1007/978-3-319-10578-9_23
20. Simonyan, K., Zisserman, A.: Very deep convolutional networks for large-scale image recognition. In: ICLR (2014)
21. Zeiler, M.D., Fergus, R.: Visualizing and understanding convolutional networks. In: Fleet, D., Pajdla, T., Schiele, B., Tuytelaars, T. (eds.) ECCV 2014. LNCS, vol. 8689, pp. 818–833. Springer, Cham (2014). doi:10.1007/978-3-319-10590-1_53
22. BI-RADS. https://en.wikipedia.org/wiki/BI-RADS

Modeling the Intra-class Variability for Liver Lesion Detection Using a Multi-class Patch-Based CNN

Maayan Frid-Adar[1(✉)], Idit Diamant[1], Eyal Klang[2], Michal Amitai[2], Jacob Goldberger[3], and Hayit Greenspan[1]

[1] Department of Biomedical Engineering, Faculty of Engineering, Tel Aviv University, Tel Aviv, Israel
maayanfrid@mail.tau.ac.il, hayit@eng.tau.ac.il
[2] Diagnostic Imaging Department, Sheba Medical Center, Tel Hashomer, Israel
[3] Faculty of Engineering, Bar-Ilan University, Ramat Gan, Israel

Abstract. Automatic detection of liver lesions in CT images poses a great challenge for researchers. In this work we present a deep learning approach that models explicitly the variability within the non-lesion class, based on prior knowledge of the data, to support an automated lesion detection system. A multi-class convolutional neural network (CNN) is proposed to categorize input image patches into sub-categories of boundary and interior patches, the decisions of which are fused to reach a binary lesion vs non-lesion decision. For validation of our system, we use CT images of 132 livers and 498 lesions. Our approach shows highly improved detection results that outperform the state-of-the-art fully convolutional network. Automated computerized tools, as shown in this work, have the potential in the future to support the radiologists towards improved detection.

Keywords: Liver lesion · Detection · Convolutional neural network · Patch-based system · Computer-aided detection

1 Introduction

Liver cancer is one of the predominant cancer types, accounting for more than 600,000 deaths each year. The number of liver tumors diagnosed throughout the world is increasing at an alarming rate. Early diagnosis and treatment is the most useful way to reduce cancer deaths. Computed tomography (CT) images are widely used for the detection and diagnosis of liver lesions. Manual detection is a time-consuming task which requires the radiologist to search through a 3D CT scan. Thus, there is an interest and need for automated analysis tools to assist clinicians in the detection of liver metastases in CT examinations.

M. Frid-Adar and I. Diamant—Equal Contributors

© Springer International Publishing AG 2017
G. Wu et al. (Eds.): Patch-MI 2017, LNCS 10530, pp. 129–137, 2017.
DOI: 10.1007/978-3-319-67434-6_15

Automatic liver lesion detection is a very challenging, clinically relevant task due to the substantial lesion appearance variation within and between patients (in size, shape, texture, contrast enhancement). In detection, both small and large lesions are weighed similarly. This is in contrast with a segmentation task that can miss small lesions and still get a high score.

This research problem has attracted much attention in recent years. The MICCAI 2008 Grand Challenge [3] provided a good overview of possible approaches mainly for segmentation. The winner of the challenge [6] used the AdaBoost classifier to separate liver lesions from normal liver tissue based on several local image features. In more recent works, deep learning [4,5,7] was applied for liver lesion detection using fully convolutional networks (FCN) [1,2]. The FCN system presented in [1] showed high detection results with TPR of 88% and 0.74 FP per liver.

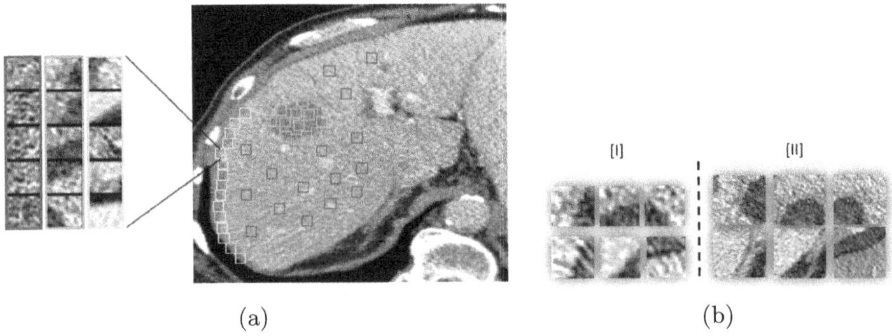

(a) (b)

Fig. 1. (a) Liver patch examples: lesion (blue), normal-interior (red) and normal-boundary (yellow); (b) Patch size 20×20 [I] and patch size 50×50 [II]. Top row: lesion boundary patch examples; Bottom row: liver boundary patch examples. (Color figure online)

A deep learning approach provides a highly non-linear data representation of a given feature x, denoted by $h(x)$. However, at the final softmax layer, the decision is a linear function of h (it is exactly a logistic regression classifier). Thus, even in the most sophisticated neural network, the normal or lesion binary decision is performed by a linear classifier that is applied to $h(x)$. In many cases the data associated with each label is not homogeneous and is organized in clusters which have different characteristics and appearance. For example, the non-lesion patches might look different given that they either located in the liver interior or in the liver boundary. In such cases a linear decision provided by the soft-max layer is not capable to handle the complex class structure.

The novelty of this study is to model the solution to the task and divide the data to sub-categories correctly with specific medical task expertise. We demonstrate this idea by modeling the intra-class variability of the non-lesion category using a Multi-class patch-based CNN system that allocates several network classes for a single medical decision. This small modification of the standard network architecture, provides a mean for modeling the within-class variability, yields a significant improvement over state-of-the-art results. Comparisons were done with state-of-the-art patch-based CNN as well as FCN. A description of the proposed architecture is presented in Sect. 2. Experiments and results are shown in Sect. 3, followed by concluding remarks in Sect. 4.

2 Multi-class Patch-Based CNN System

We propose a system for lesion detection, which is based on localized patch classification into lesion vs non-lesion categories. Patches are an important representation to address the data limitation challenge, critical for modeling small and rare events such as lesions. Figure 1a shows examples of lesion patches, including lesion-boundary patches (shown blue zoomed-in), as well as patches from the non-lesion category, which include both normal-interior patches (red) and normal-boundary patches (yellow). As can be seen in Fig. 1b[I], liver boundary and lesion boundary areas may look alike and are difficult to distinguish when using small patches. When using a larger size window, a clearer distinction between the two categories is possible, as seen in Fig. 1b[II]. This motivated us to use two different scales (patch-sizes) within the proposed system to capture both the local fine details and the more global spatial information.

We note that the normal-interior patches and the normal-boundary patches have a distinct appearance, yet both comprise the non-lesion category. We therefore propose a solution that is aware of this intra-class variability and allocates a different label (with different soft-max parameters) for the interior and boundary patches. Since eventually we are only interested in lesion/non-lesion decision, at test time we merge the non-lesion classes by summing-up their probabilities into a single probability of a non-lesion.

2.1 Patch Extraction

Patches are extracted from 2D liver CT scans with an expert marking for the lesions. The liver area can be segmented automatically or by an expert. The patches are labeled with their corresponding class $k \in \{$lesion, normal-interior, normal-boundary$\}$, automatically, according to their relative position to the boundary. The patches are extracted around each pixel in two fields-of-view (FOV) of size 20×20 pixels and 50×50 pixels. The patches contain localized information as well as spatial context. All patches are resized to 32×32 pixels to fit the input image size of our multi-class CNN architecture.

The amount of patches in the normal-interior class is much larger than the number of patches in other classes. Therefore, the patches are sampled randomly to balance the training set. Data augmentation is applied to enrich the lesion class by flipping {right,left} and rotating in $[5, 130, 300]$ angles. Patches are sampled with overlap using a 2-pixel step size between patch centers.

All patches are normalized as follows: during training, the mean liver intensity was calculated on the training set: $I_{mean} = \frac{1}{N}\sum_j p(x_j, y_j)$ where N is the number of pixels in the liver area. During the testing phase, in order to obtain uniform mean liver intensity in all livers, we shifted the patches intensities such that each test liver will have a mean intensity value equal I_{mean} (mean liver intensity of training set).

2.2 System Architecture

We propose a multi-class patch-based CNN, as shown in Fig. 2. The architecture of the network consists of 4 convolutional (conv.) layers and 3 pooling layers (one max-pooling and two avg-pooling). Each conv. layer is followed by a ReLU activation function. The network has approx. 0.15 million parameters.

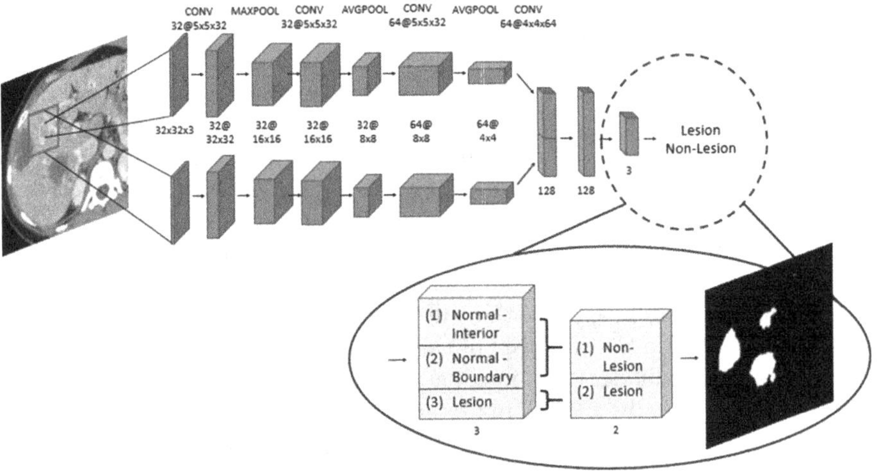

Fig. 2. The Parallel multi-class CNN architecture: combining multi-class (to handle within class variability) and multi-scale (to handle inter-class similarity).

Our system receives input patches in two FOVs around each pixel. The scaled patches are analyzed in parallel using two different networks that are late fused in the last fully-connected layer. The last layer is a softmax classifier that calculates the probabilities of the patch (which correspond to the probabilities of the center pixel) for each class. The probabilities are retrieved using multinomial logistic regression:

$$p(y = k|x) = \frac{\exp(S_k)}{\sum_j \exp(S_j)} \tag{1}$$

where k is the class label, $S_k = w_k^T h(x) + b_k$ is the score or the unnormalized log probability of class k given the non-linear representation $h(x)$.

At the testing stage, the lesion detection map is generated for the interior area of the liver by replacing each pixel with its corresponding patch probability for the lesion category. All normal sub-category probabilities are summarized into one non-lesion class probability:

$$p_{\text{non-lesion}} = p_{\text{normal-boundary}} + p_{\text{normal-interior}} \tag{2}$$

We threshold the lesion detection probability map to obtain a binary detection map. Herein, we term the network described above as the *Parallel multi-class CNN.*

We also implemented another multi-class approach which is based on *hierarchical binary-class* CNNs. It is implemented by splitting the three category classification task into two steps. The first step generates a map of lesion candidates by using binary classification of lesion and non-lesion areas ('lesion detector'). The second step performs false-positive reduction using a binary-class CNN which is trained to classify between lesion and non-lesion using only normal patches located at the liver boundary and lesion patches located anywhere in the liver. This CNN is applied to the lesion candidates which were obtained from the output of the first step. We implemented the lesion detector using a binary-class CNN.

2.3 Training Protocol

In order to train our multi-class CNN we minimize the cross-entropy loss:

$$L_i = -\log p(y_i|x_i) = -(S(y_i) - \log \sum_j \exp(S_j)), \qquad L = \frac{1}{N}\sum_{i=1}^{N} L_i \quad (3)$$

where y_i is the ground truth label of input x_i and $S(y_i)$ is its corresponding score. The CNN was trained using 140,000 patches for each class. The networks were trained on a NVIDIA GeForce GTX 980 Ti GPU and implemented using MatConvNet deep learning framework [8]. We tried two initialization scenarios for the parameters of the conv. layers: one using random Gaussian distributions ("trained from scratch") and one using transfer learning from the Cifar-10 dataset ("fine-tuned" system). When performing transfer learning, initialization of each channel is pretrained on Cifar-10 dataset separately and the joint fully-connected layers are initialized randomly. For random initialization (training from scratch) we use learning rate of 0.0001 for the first 30 epochs and decreasing by 1/10 each 10 epochs with total of 50 epochs. Weights are initialized randomly and updated using mini-batches of 128 examples and stochastic gradient descent optimization. Weight decay was chosen to be 0.0001 with momentum of 0.9. When using transfer learning, convolution layers are initialized with Cifar-10 pre-trained network and learning rate is set to zero. The two last joint fully-connected layers are initialized randomly with learning rate of 1.

3 Experiments and Results

We evaluated our multi-class CNN system on a liver metastases dataset from Sheba Medical Center. Cases were acquired between 2009 and 2014 using different CT scanners with 0.71–1.17 mm pixel spacing and 1.25–5.0 mm slice thickness. Cases were collected with approval of the institutions Institutional Review Board. The dataset includes 132 2D liver CT scans with overall of 498 metastases in various shapes, contrast and sizes (5.0–121.0 mm) where each liver contains one or multiple (1–10) lesions. Cases were selected and marked by an expert radiologist. Images were resized to a fixed pixel spacing of 0.71 mm.

3.1 Comparison to State-of-the-Art

We first evaluated our proposed approach on the relatively small dataset which was used in [1] for comparison purposes. This dataset includes 20 patients and contains 43 CT liver scans with overall of 68 metastases, where each liver contains 1–3 lesions. Evaluation was performed with 3-fold cross-validation with case separation at the patient level.

Table 1 shows detection performance comparison of our multi-class system to alternative architectures. We compared our system to the classical detection approach which uses only two classes, lesion and normal tissue, implemented with a *binary-class CNN*. Results show that our Multi-class approach achieves higher detection performance than using a binary-class CNN. Moreover, our proposed system improves over the state-of-the-art FCN system (which was presented in MICCAI 2016 Workshop [1]). Note that the 3-slice FCN includes also two neighboring slices which we did not use in our implementation.

Table 1. Lesion detection performance evaluation: 43 liver dataset; comparison to state-of-the-art [1].

Method	TPR	FPC
Parallel multi-class CNN	98.4%	1.0
Hierarchical multi-class CNN	98.4%	0.9
Binary-class CNN	95.2%	1.0
FCN (3 slices) [1]	88.0%	0.74
FCN [1]	85.0%	1.1

We note that we obtained comparable results for the hierarchical and parallel multi-class CNNs. The advantage of the parallel scheme is that there is only a single network we need to train.

Detection results can be seen in Fig. 3. The information retained from the sub-categories improves the detection performance and the robustness of the system as compared to the binary-class implementation. It reduces the false-positives in the normal tissue mainly at the liver boundary but also in the interior area of the liver.

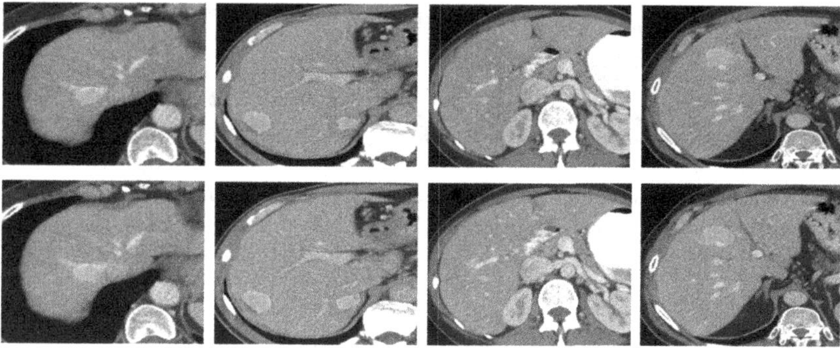

Fig. 3. Examples of lesion detection results. First row: Parallel multi-class CNN. Second row: Binary-class CNN. TP marked in green, FP in red and FN in blue. (Color figure online)

3.2 Detection Performance Evaluation

We next evaluated the proposed method on a larger dataset that extended the first to include additional variability overall, from (institution name withheld). Evaluation was performed on the 132 livers with 2-fold cross-validation. Table 2 shows comparison results of our proposed method to other CNN-based systems. Detection results are shown for the entire dataset, as well as for a subset of the larger lesions >10 mm, which are the ones mostly recorded by the radiologists and require immediate care. When applied to all lesion sizes, our proposed method resulted in 85.9% TPR and 1.9 FP per liver (FPC) while the binary-class CNN resulted in 80% TPR with 2.8 FPC.

Table 2. Lesion detection performance evaluation: 132 liver dataset.

Method	All lesion sizes		lesions >10 mm	
	TPR	FPC	TPR	FPC
Parallel multi-class CNN	85.9%	1.9	93.0%	1.5
Hierarchical multi-class CNN	86.8%	1.9	91.8%	1.5
Binary-class CNN	80.0%	2.8	70.0%	1.9

Our multi-class hierarchical approach resulted in similar performance of 86.8% TPR with 1.9 FPC. Using transfer learning for this task (see Sect. 2.2) was not as successful as training from scratch (obtaining 82.8% TPR with 2.54 FPC when applied on all lesion sizes). The detection performance is higher when excluding small lesions (<10 mm), with 93.0% TPR and 1.5 FPC using our parallel multi-class system and 91.8% TPR with 1.56 FPC using our Hierarchical approach. Figure 4 shows detection examples, demonstrating the ability of our system to detect a variety of lesion sizes. We emphasize that the only difference

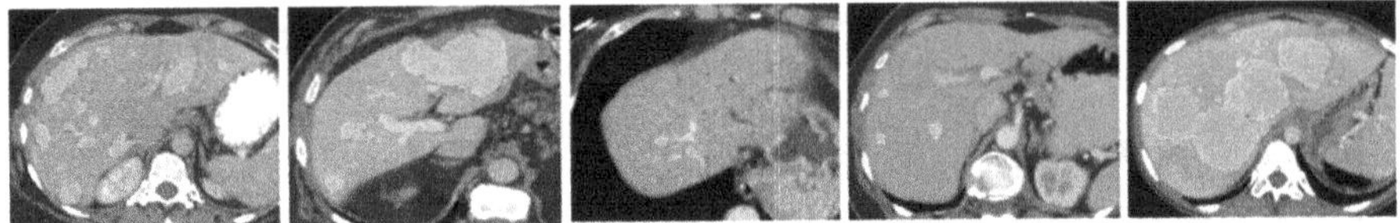

Fig. 4. Examples of lesion detection results showing the variability in lesions size, location and shape. TP marked in green, FP in red and FN in blue. (Color figure online)

between the binary-class and the multi-class networks shown in Table 2 is the multi-class description of the non-lesion patches at the final softmax layer of the multi-class network. As can be seen from Table 2, this small network architecture difference yields a huge performance difference.

4 Conclusions

We presented a multi-class patch-based CNN architecture for liver lesion detection in CT images. Our method takes into account the variability of the normal liver tissue and the spatial information retrieved using different scales of view. We showed that separating the inhomogeneous normal class to sub-categories improves detection performance as compared to a binary-class implementation. Our approach outperformed the state-of-the-art method which is based on a fully convolutional network. In future work we plan to focus on the lesion class and explore its separation into a dual category: lesion interior and lesion boundary classes, towards improved lesion segmentation. Our approach may generalize to additional medical detection applications. Automated computerized tools, as shown in this work, have the potential in the future to support the radiologists towards improved detection.

References

1. Ben-Cohen, A., Diamant, I., Klang, E., Amitai, M., Greenspan, H.: Fully convolutional network for liver segmentation and lesions detection. In: Carneiro, G., et al. (eds.) LABELS/DLMIA -2016. LNCS, vol. 10008, pp. 77–85. Springer, Cham (2016). doi:10.1007/978-3-319-46976-8_9
2. Christ, P.F., et al.: Automatic liver and lesion segmentation in CT using cascaded fully convolutional neural networks and 3D conditional random fields. In: Ourselin, S., Joskowicz, L., Sabuncu, M.R., Unal, G., Wells, W. (eds.) MICCAI 2016. LNCS, vol. 9901, pp. 415–423. Springer, Cham (2016). doi:10.1007/978-3-319-46723-8_48
3. Deng, X., Du, G.: Editorial: 3D segmentation in the clinic: a grand challenge ii-liver tumor segmentation. In: MICCAI Workshop (2008)
4. Greenspan, H., van Ginneken, B., Summers, R.: Guest editorial deep learning in medical imaging: overview and future promise of an exciting new technique. IEEE Trans. Med. Imaging **35**, 1153–1159 (2016)

5. Setio, A.A.A., et al.: Pulmonary nodule detection in CT images: false positive reduction using multi-view convolutional networks. IEEE Trans. Med. Imaging **35**(5), 1160–1169 (2016)
6. Shimizu, A., et al.: Ensemble segmentation using AdaBoost with application to liver lesion extraction from a ct volume. In: Proceedings of Medical Imaging Computing Computer Assisted Intervention Workshop on 3D Segmentation in the Clinic: A Grand Challenge II (2008)
7. Shin, H.C., et al.: Deep convolutional neural networks for computer-aided detection: CNN architectures, dataset characteristics and transfer learning. IEEE Trans. Med. Imaging **35**(5), 1285–1298 (2016)
8. Vedaldi, A., Lenc, K.: Matconvnet: convolutional neural networks for matlab. In: Proceedings of the 23rd Annual ACM Conference on Multimedia Conference, pp. 689–692 (2015)

Multiple Sclerosis Lesion Segmentation Using Joint Label Fusion

Mengjin Dong[1(✉)], Ipek Oguz[1], Nagesh Subbana[1], Peter Calabresi[2], Russell T. Shinohara[3], and Paul Yushkevich[1]

[1] Penn Image Computing and Science Lab, University of Pennsylvania, Philadelphia, PA, USA
mengjin@seas.upenn.edu
[2] The Johns Hopkins Calabresi Lab, Johns Hopkins University, Baltimore, MD, USA
[3] Center for Clinical Epidemiology and Biostatistics, University of Pennsylvania, Philadelphia, PA, USA

Abstract. This paper adapts the joint label fusion (JLF) multi-atlas image segmentation algorithm to the problem of multiple sclerosis (MS) lesion segmentation in multi-modal MRI. Conventionally, JLF requires a set of atlas images to be co-registered to the target image using deformable registration. However, given the variable spatial distribution of lesions in the brain, whole-brain deformable registration is unlikely to line up lesions between atlases and the target image. As a solution, we propose to first pre-segment the target image using an intensity regression based technique, yielding a set of "candidate" lesions. Each "candidate" lesion is then matched to a set of similar lesions in the atlas based on location and size; and deformable registration and JLF are applied at the level of the "candidate" lesion. The approach is evaluated on a dataset of 74 subjects with MS and shown to improve Dice similarity coefficient with reference manual segmentation by 12% over intensity regression technique.

1 Introduction

Multiple sclerosis (MS) is a degenerative disease of the central nervous system in which the axonal myelin sheath is damaged due to an autoimmune reaction. There is no cure for MS; however, early detection and tracking of the lesions play a vital part in the clinical management of the disease. The burden of the disease (volume of lesions) and the number of lesions in the brain are important metrics in tracking disease and the efficacy of therap.

Manual segmentation of MS lesions is costly and suffers from low reliability due to differences between experts [6]. Consequently, automatic segmentation of lesions using multiple MRI modalities is the preferred approach to quantifying lesion burden. Automatic segmentation of lesions is complicated by variability in the shape, size and position of MS lesions and the differences in the apparent extent of lesions across different MRI modalities. Many techniques for automatic MS lesion segmentation have been proposed and evaluated, as reviewed in [8].

© Springer International Publishing AG 2017
G. Wu et al. (Eds.): Patch-MI 2017, LNCS 10530, pp. 138–145, 2017.
DOI: 10.1007/978-3-319-67434-6_16

The largest class of techniques performs statistical inference on image intensity using unsupervised or supervised approaches, and frequently incorporating spatial priors such as Markov random fields; examples include [4,6,11–14].

Recently, patch-based multi-atlas segmentation techniques have been applied to MS lesion segmentation with considerable success [5,9,10]. These methods use large libraries of patches extracted from expert-annotated atlases to match candidate patches in the target image. The advantage of this approach is that it incorporates anatomical context into the segmentation decision: the decision to assign a voxel a label of lesion or non-lesion is based not only on voxel intensity characteristics but on the intensity and texture of the surrounding region. However, a limitation is that they are restrictive in terms of the transformations that atlas patches may undergo when matching the target image. For example, the atlas and the target image may contain a periventricular lesion of similar appearance, but if the ventricle is thin in the atlas and enlarged in the target, the patch similarity metric may be low. Allowing atlas patches to deform, as is proposed in this paper, may improve the segmentation of the target lesion.

Multi-atlas label fusion (MALF) is an approach that a set of expert-labeled atlas images are matched to the target image – typically using non-linear registration – and segmentations from deformed atlas images are fused into a consensus segmentation of the target image [7]. Effective label fusion techniques weigh atlases based on local intensity similarity to the target image [7]. In particular, joint label fusion (JLF) assigns spatially varying atlas weights in a way that accounts for error correlations between pairs of atlases, achieving excellent performance in brain structure segmentation [15]. However, conventional MALF is ill-suited for MS lesion segmentation since whole-brain registration is unlikely to match MS lesions between individuals due to variability in lesion location and extent. In this paper, we adapt JLF to MS lesion segmentation by performing non-linear registration on a regional, rather than whole-brain level. The approach consists of three components:

1. Pre-segmentation of the target image into "candidate" lesions using the OASIS intensity-based technique [13]. For each "candidate" lesion, a region of interest (ROI) is extracted from the MRI. Very large candidate lesions are broken up into smaller overlapping ROIs.
2. Selection of a subset of anatomically similar atlas ROIs for each target "candidate" lesion ROI.
3. Non-linear registration of atlas ROIs to the target ROI and JLF-based segmentation of the target ROI.

These components are detailed below and an evaluation of the proposed approach is carried out in a set of 74 multicontrast MRI scans of patients with MS. The results indicate that regional JLF segmentation improves accuracy relative to manual segmentation over intensity-based segmentation alone. To our knowledge, this is the first application of MALF with deformable registration to the problem of MS lesion segmentation.

2 Materials and Methods

2.1 Imaging Data

Analysis is carried out in a cross-sectional dataset of 3 tesla T1-weighted and FLAIR MRI acquired in 94 MS patients. The generation of OASIS also uses T2-weighted and PD-weighted. MS lesions were segmented manually in all images by a trained expert with 10+ years of experience. MRI volumes were skull stripped via the algorithm SPECTRE and then bias field corrected using the N3 algorithm. FLAIR volumes were rigidly aligned to the T1-weighted MRI. Figure 1 shows an example of the image data.

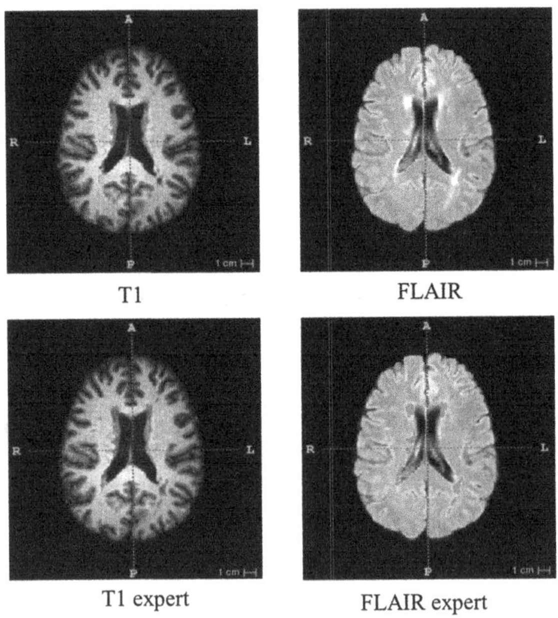

Fig. 1. T1-weighted and FLAIR MRI (axial plane) for one subject, with expert segmentation superimposed in the bottom row.

2.2 Lesion Pre-segmentation

The goal of pre-segmentation is to produce a pool of "candidate" lesions that includes most of the "true" lesions in the target image but may also include false positives. In subsequent steps, MALF is used to refine this segmentation, with the goal of refining lesion boundaries and removing false positives. Pre-segmentation is produced using the OASIS approach, which fits a logistic regression model to the normalized T1 and FLAIR MRI intensity of lesion and non-lesion voxels in the training set [13]. Thresholding this probability map at a given level ρ gives a binary segmentation of the lesions. Sweeney et al. report the sensitivity and specificity of OASIS for different levels of ρ [13]. OASIS was trained on 20 of the 94 subjects' data and applied to the remaining 74 subjects. Based on previous experience with the OASIS method and visual inspection of the data in the training set, we adopted a threshold of $\rho = 0.25$. The 20-subject OASIS training data was not used in subsequent experiments.

Candidate lesions are obtained by splitting the binary OASIS output into connected components. Components smaller than 3 voxels were discarded. Additionally, we broke up large components into separate sub-components, because in some subjects periventricular lesions yield a single connected component and in others they yield several connected components, and the matching strategy discussed below is based on global morphological features (size, location) that match up poorly between contiguous and split candidate periventricular lesions. To split connected components we use the SLIC supervoxel algorithm [1] with the approximate supervoxel size of $\frac{1}{10}$ of the image dimensions. Each candidate lesion (or sub-lesion) was then padded by 10 voxels on each side, yielding a set of rectilinear ROIs. Corresponding ROIs were extracted from the FLAIR and T1-weighted images. We refer to these as "lesion ROIs".

2.3 MALF Approach and Cross-Validation Overview

The dataset of 74 subjects processed by OASIS was randomly split into five training/testing folds with 59 training image and 15 test images (the fifth fold had 60 training and 14 testing images). All subsequent analysis was repeated independently for each fold. Each candidate lesion ROI in each training image of each fold was processed in parallel. For each such "target" lesion ROI, we first select a set of 50 suitable lesion ROIs from the training subset (Atlas Selection) and then perform MALF segmentation using these 50 lesion ROIs as atlases. These steps are described below.

2.4 Atlas Selection

Atlas selection is necessary because the total number of lesion ROIs in the training subset is too large (order of 1000) and most lesion ROIs are contextually different from a given target lesion. To perform atlas selection, we compare each OASIS-extracted candidate lesion in the training subset to target candidate lesion based on three factors: (1) lesion size (after splitting by SLIC algorithm); (2) distance from the lesion center to the lateral ventricles; (3) location of the closest point on the lateral ventricles. To compute (2) and (3), we register each subject's T1-weighted MRI to a whole-brain template, and warp a surface mesh representation of the ventricles defined in template space into the subject's space. For each lesion i, we then find a vertex on the ventricle surface $\mathbf{x}_v^i$ that is closest to the lesion center $\mathbf{x}_c^i$. Given two lesions i and j, we compute the triple of similarity metrics,

$$\left\{ \left|\log\left(\frac{V_i}{V_j}\right)\right|, \left|\frac{|\mathbf{x}_v^i - \mathbf{x}_c^i|}{\sqrt[3]{V_i^{\mathrm{TB}} - V_i^{\mathrm{LV}}}} - \frac{|\mathbf{x}_v^j - \mathbf{x}_c^j|}{\sqrt[3]{V_j^{\mathrm{TB}} - V_j^{\mathrm{LV}}}}\right|, d_v(\mathbf{x}_v^i, \mathbf{x}_v^j) \right\},$$

where V_i is the volume of the lesion i, V_i^{TB} is the total brain volume, V_i^{LV} is the lateral ventricle volume, and $d_v(\mathbf{x}_v^i, \mathbf{x}_v^j)$ is the geodesic distance between ventricle mesh vertices corresponding to $\mathbf{x}_v^i$ and $\mathbf{x}_v^j$ in template space. Lesions are considered contextually similar if the three metrics are low. Since the metrics have different units, for a given target lesion i, we rank all training lesions separately on each metric, resulting in a triple of rank values. The 50 training lesions with the smallest mean rank value are "atlases" for segmenting the target lesion.

The above atlas selection strategy is motivated by the importance of the ventricles in providing context for MS lesion segmentation. Many MS lesions are adjacent to the ventricles (periventricular) and the shape, size and appearance is likely to be similar at the same location relative to the ventricles. The ranking strategy may select atlases that not very similar to the target ROI, but the JLF method will weight less on them.

2.5 Joint Label Fusion

Given a target lesion ROI and a set of 50 training lesion ROIs obtained by atlas selection, the standard JLF approach is employed. Each atlas lesion ROI is registered to the target ROI using a greedy diffeomorphic registration method [3]. Registration is initialized by matching the centers of mass of the candidate lesions between the atlas and target ROIs. Deformable registration maximizes the local cross-correlation metric with a $9 \times 9 \times 9$ voxel window and is regularized by Gaussian smoothing of the deformation field at each iteration, as in [2]. The T1-weighted and FLAIR images contribute equally to the metric computation.

After registration, the atlas FLAIR and T1-weighted ROIs are resliced into the target image space. The corresponding expert segmentation is also warped to target image space (although some atlas ROIs may be false positives and contain empty expert segmentations). The warped images and segmentations are input to the JLF algorithm [15], which produces a spatially varying voting weight map $w_i(\mathbf{x})$ for each atlas i. To compute the weights $\{w_i\}$ at a voxel $\mathbf{x}$, the total expected segmentation error is minimized with respect to $\{w_i\}$. The total segmentation error is expressed as pairwise expected joint segmentation errors for all pairs of atlases $\{i, j\}$. The latter is approximated by considering patch similarities between atlases i and j and the target image, as described in [15].

3 Results

Segmentation was run on a multi-CPU cluster with 30 parallel processes each using two cores. For 15-image test set, segmentation required about an hour, with most time spent in deformable registration and JLF computation.

Figure 2 shows an example of the segmentation by the proposed method, compared with segmentation by OASIS alone and expert manual segmentation.

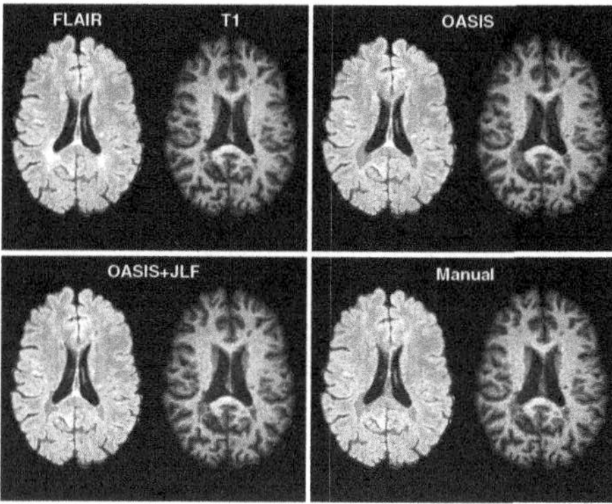

Fig. 2. An example dataset with segmentations produced by OASIS, the proposed method (OASIS+JLF) and manually.

Table 1 reports, for each cross-validation fold, the mean Dice similarity coefficient between the expert segmentation and the automatic segmentations obtained by OASIS alone and the proposed method, with OASIS threshold $\rho = 0.25$. The mean Dice coefficient across all five folds was 0.52 ± 0.22 for OASIS and 0.59 ± 0.19 for the proposed method, corresponding to roughly 12% improvement. The 95% confidence interval on the improvement in Dice coefficient is $(0.04, 0.09)$, i.e., the improvement is highly significant.

Table 1. The Dice similarity coefficients of the five-fold cross-validation for JLF against the expert segmentations and the corresponding OASIS values on each fold with OASIS threshold $\rho = 0.25$.

Technique	Fold 1	Fold 2	Fold 3	Fold 4	Fold 5	Average
OASIS	0.5160	0.5479	0.5147	0.4855	0.5467	0.5218
JLF	0.5827	0.6221	0.5770	0.5433	0.6062	0.5860

We also observed that segmentation performance varies by the total lesion burden in each subject (i.e., total volume of all expert-segmented lesions). Figure 3 shows a scatter plot of OASIS vs. JLF Dice coefficient for different testing subjects, with the total lesion burden indicated for each subject. Overall, Dice coefficient is higher in subjects with greater lesion burden. The improvement from JLF is more notable in subjects with lesser lesion burden, suggesting that JLF improves the segmentation of small lesions more than large lesions.

Modulating the OASIS threshold ρ can increase the number and size of candidate lesions. Values of ρ below 0.25 should result in over-segmentation of the lesions, on average; and it is possible that by removing false positives, JLF would perform better for smaller values of ρ than the optimal OASIS threshold. Figure 4 plots the Dice coefficient for OASIS and JLF for different values of ρ between 0.2

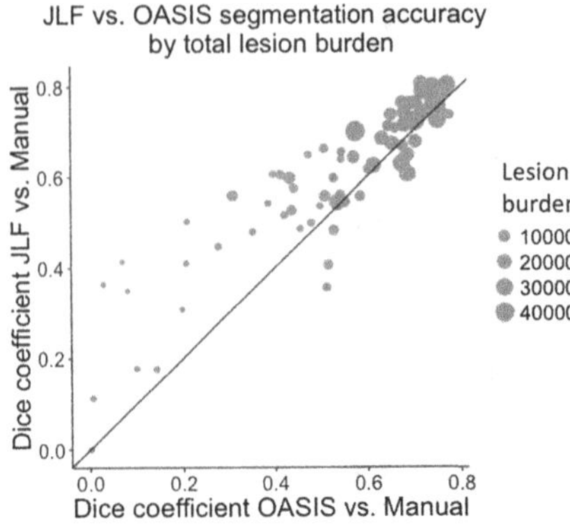

Fig. 3. Comparison of JLF vs OASIS segmentation accuracy by total lesion burden.

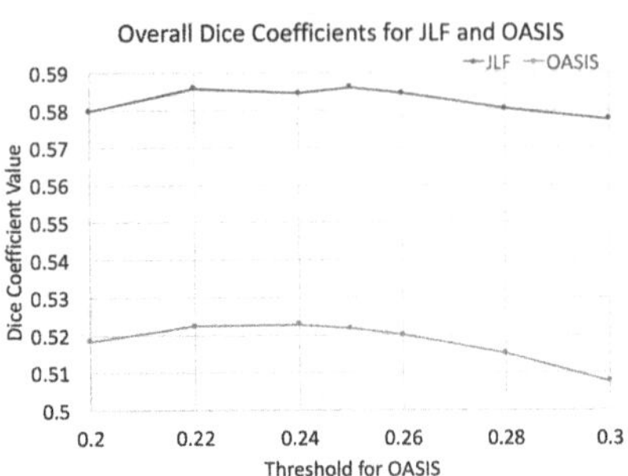

Fig. 4. Comparison of Dice similarity coefficients for OASIS and JLF methods using different OASIS thresholds ρ. Average Dice coefficient across all five folds is plotted.

and 0.3. However, surprisingly, there is no apparent advantage to using smaller threshold values for JLF accuracy.

4 Conclusion

We proposed an approach for MS lesion segmentation that behaves as a wrapper around an intensity-based lesion segmentation technique (OASIS) and performs multi-atlas segmentation separately for each candidate lesion ROI identified by the intensity-based technique. The approach is the first application of the joint label fusion algorithm to MS lesion segmentation. The addition of the JLF improves MS lesion segmentation performance by 12% over OASIS, which is considered a state of the art technique. Future work will focus on using other approaches to generate candidate lesions, comparisons on grand challenge data, and extensions to 4D lesion modeling.

Acknowledgments. This work was supported, in part, by the NIH grants NIBIB R01EB017255, NINDS R01NS082347, NINDS R01NS085211, NINDS R21NS093349, NINDS R01NS094456.

References

1. Achanta, R., Shaji, A., Smith, K., Lucchi, A., Fua, P., Süsstrunk, S.: SLIC superpixels compared to state-of-the-art superpixel methods. IEEE Trans. Pattern Anal. Mach. Intell. **34**(11), 2274–2282 (2012)
2. Avants, B.B., Epstein, C.L., Grossman, M., Gee, J.C.: Symmetric diffeomorphic image registration with cross-correlation: evaluating automated labeling of elderly and neurodegenerative brain. Med. Image Anal. **12**(1), 26–41 (2008)
3. Avants, B., Gee, J.C.: Geodesic estimation for large deformation anatomical shape averaging and interpolation. Neuroimage **23**(Suppl. 1), S139–S150 (2004)

4. Freifeld, O., Greenspan, H., Goldberger, J.: Multiple sclerosis lesion detection using constrained GMM and curve evolution. Int. J. Biomed. Imaging **2009**, 715124 (2009)
5. Guizard, N., Coupé, P., Fonov, V.S., Manjón, J.V., Arnold, D.L., Collins, D.L.: Rotation-invariant multi-contrast non-local means for MS lesion segmentation. Neuroimage Clin. **8**, 376–389 (2015)
6. Harmouche, R., Subbanna, N.K., Collins, D.L., Arnold, D.L., Arbel, T.: Probabilistic multiple sclerosis lesion classification based on modeling regional intensity variability and local neighborhood information. IEEE Trans. Biomed. Eng. **62**(5), 1281–1292 (2015)
7. Iglesias, J.E., Sabuncu, M.R.: Multi-atlas segmentation of biomedical images: a survey. Med. Image Anal. **24**(1), 205–219 (2015)
8. Lladó, X., Oliver, A., Cabezas, M., Freixenet, J., Vilanova, J.C., Quiles, A., Valls, L., Ramió-Torrentà, L., Rovira, A.: Segmentation of multiple sclerosis lesions in brain MRI: a review of automated approaches. Inf. Sci. **186**(1), 164–185 (2012)
9. Mechrez, R., Goldberger, J., Greenspan, H.: Patch-based segmentation with spatial consistency: application to ms lesions in brain MRI. J. Biomed. Imaging **2016**, 3 (2016)
10. Roy, S., He, Q., Carass, A., Jog, A., Cuzzocreo, J.L., Reich, D.S., Prince, J., Pham, D.: Example based lesion segmentation. In: SPIE Medical Imaging, p. 90341Y. International Society for Optics and Photonics (2014)
11. Schmidt, P., Gaser, C., Arsic, M., Buck, D., Förschler, A., Berthele, A., Hoshi, M., Ilg, R., Schmid, V.J., Zimmer, C., Hemmer, B., Mühlau, M.: An automated tool for detection of flair-hyperintense white-matter lesions in multiple sclerosis. Neuroimage **59**(4), 3774–3783 (2012)
12. Shiee, N., Bazin, P.L., Ozturk, A., Reich, D.S., Calabresi, P.A., Pham, D.L.: A topology-preserving approach to the segmentation of brain images with multiple sclerosis lesions. Neuroimage **49**(2), 1524–1535 (2010)
13. Sweeney, E.M., Shinohara, R.T., Shiee, N., Mateen, F.J., Chudgar, A.A., Cuzzocreo, J.L., Calabresi, P.A., Pham, D.L., Reich, D.S., Crainiceanu, C.M.: OASIS is automated statistical inference for segmentation, with applications to multiple sclerosis lesion segmentation in MRI. NeuroImage: Clin. **2**, 402–413 (2013)
14. Van Leemput, K., Maes, F., Vandermeulen, D., Colchester, A., Suetens, P.: Automated segmentation of multiple sclerosis lesions by model outlier detection. IEEE Trans. Med. Imaging **20**(8), 677–688 (2001)
15. Wang, H., Suh, J.W., Das, S.R., Pluta, J.B., Craige, C., Yushkevich, P.A.: Multi-atlas segmentation with joint label fusion. IEEE Trans. Pattern Anal. Mach. Intell. **35**(3), 611–623 (2013)

Classification, Retrieval

Deep Multimodal Case–Based Retrieval for Large Histopathology Datasets

Oscar Jimenez-del-Toro[1,2(✉)], Sebastian Otálora[1,2], Manfredo Atzori[1], and Henning Müller[1,2]

[1] University of Geneva (UNIGE), Geneva, Switzerland
oscar.jimenez@hevs.ch
[2] University of Applied Sciences Western Switzerland (HES-SO), Sierre, Switzerland

Abstract. The current gold standard for interpreting patient tissue samples is the visual inspection of whole–slide histopathology images (WSIs) by pathologists. They generate a pathology report describing the main findings relevant for diagnosis and treatment planning. Searching for similar cases through repositories for differential diagnosis is often not done due to a lack of efficient strategies for medical case–based retrieval. A patch–based multimodal retrieval strategy that retrieves similar pathology cases from a large data set fusing both visual and text information is explained in this paper. By fine–tuning a deep convolutional neural network an automatic representation is obtained for the visual content of weakly annotated WSIs (using only a global cancer score and no manual annotations). The pathology text report is embedded into a category vector of the pathology terms also in a non–supervised approach. A publicly available data set of 267 prostate adenocarcinoma cases with their WSIs and corresponding pathology reports was used to train and evaluate each modality of the retrieval method. A MAP (Mean Average Precision) of 0.54 was obtained with the multimodal method in a previously unseen test set. The proposed retrieval system can help in differential diagnosis of tissue samples and during the training of pathologists, exploiting the large amount of pathology data already existing digital hospital repositories.

1 Introduction

Health professionals often take decisions based on previously acquired textbook knowledge and their personal experience but rarely search for past cases to reinforce their medical assessment. Retrieval systems are developed to better exploit the large amount of digital medical data contained in hospital repositories for clinical decision support [1]. In retrieval systems, a query can be performed using text information, images or both (multimodal), resulting in a list of relevant cases ranked according to their similarity with the query case [2]. The integration of these systems into the clinical workflow remains a challenge [3].

In [4], a multimodal radiology case–based retrieval benchmark was reviewed. The cases included radiologic RadLex terms automatically extracted from radiology reports and 3D patient scans. Image retrieval systems have also been proposed in the growing field of digital pathology [5–7]. Nevertheless, multimodal

© Springer International Publishing AG 2017
G. Wu et al. (Eds.): Patch-MI 2017, LNCS 10530, pp. 149–157, 2017.
DOI: 10.1007/978-3-319-67434-6_17

case–based retrieval strategies for histopathology are rare, even though they could be a helpful tool for pathologists during training and to perform differential diagnosis. To our knowledge, only one multimodal retrieval system fusing histopathology image patches and semantics exists [5]. However, this method did not explore full pathology reports (since it was based on manual data annotations) and included only isolated image patches.

Whole Slide Image (WSI) scanning started to be applied at a large scale only recently, and a full digitization of pathology departments in hospitals will result in large scale digital WSI repositories [8]. Pathologists usually select candidate regions of interest (ROIs) in the WSIs at a low resolution and proceed to evaluate the selected regions in high–power fields. Currently available retrieval systems for histopathology are designed with either small tissue arrays, ROIs from WSIs or individual patches as visual input. To the best of our knowledge, there are no methods in literature proposed for WSI retrieval.

Hand–crafted visual features, such as texture and architecture features, are commonly used to represent images in retrieval systems [9]. In the past few years, deep learning (DL) methods have obtained a better performance for visual content description in comparison with traditional hand–crafted features in this regard [10–12]. In this paper, we propose a content–based retrieval system that uses the output features from a fine–tuned DL model, trained to classify cancer gradings in histopathology images, to represent the visual features from WSIs. An unsupervised analysis of the pathology report content was used to train the DL model and not time–consuming manual annotations from pathologists in the WSIs. This enables the reuse of already existing pathology cases for a more integral comparison of new cases to previously assessed ones. A search can in this case be a full case with WSIs and a report or only one of the two, giving several options for browsing.

2 Methods

2.1 Data Set

The Cancer Genome Atlas (TCGA) contains a large collection of digital pathology WSIs and their corresponding pathology reports [13][1]. Cases with prostate adenocarcinoma (PRAD), the second most common cancer in men, are available [14]. The Gleason grading is the standard evaluation of histopathological samples from prostate cancer patients [15]. 267 cases (WSIs and pathology reports) from prostatectomies of patients with prostate adenocarcinoma (PRAD) were included in this work, aiming at having balanced Gleason scores. The Gleason score (6–10) given to each WSI was manually obtained from the reports. The number of cases for each Gleason score were: G6 35, G7 87, G8 53, G9 83, G10 9. The cases were randomly divided as follows: 162 WSIs for training, 54 WSIs for validation and 51 WSIs for testing (approx. 60%–20%–20%). The pathology

[1] http://cancergenome.nih.gov/, as of 11 June 2017.

report length and content varied depending on the pathology center that generated them and the patient case. The hematoxylin and eosin stained WSIs do not contain any manual annotations (Fig. 1).

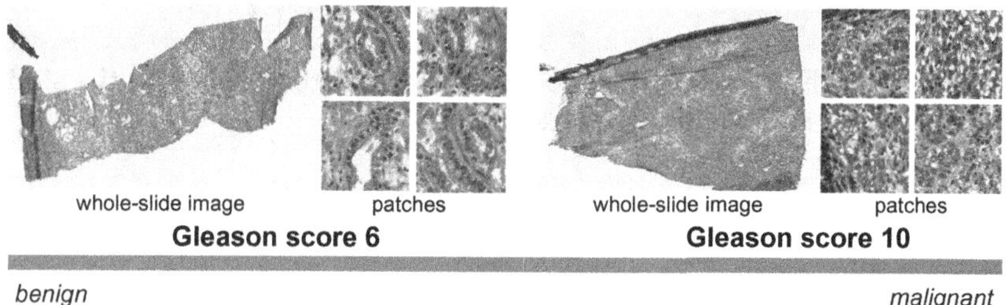

Fig. 1. Sample prostatectomy whole–slide images and patches. Far right: WSI and patches corresponding to the lowest Gleason score, G6. Far left: WSI and patches with the highest Gleason score, G10.

2.2 Whole–Slide Image Representation

A Convolutional Neural Network (CNN) is a specialized type of neural network that can learn abstract and complex representations of visual data using a large number of training samples [16]. Manually annotating WSIs in order to obtain exclusively tumor patches from the WSIs, is a time–consuming and challenging task. In [17], it was shown that a CNN can be successfully trained to classify WSIs for prostate cancer grading with a fully automatic sampling of weakly labeled patches i.e. only using the global Gleason score. A subset of 5000 random patches were initially sampled per WSI. The number of cells in tissue increases in the presence of tumors, which results in dark blue areas in the WSI due to the eosin staining of cell nuclei. The sampled patches were subsequently ranked according to the energy of the blue–ratio (BR), which is a feature that can be closely related to cell density. Only the top 2000 patches from each WSI are considered for characterizing the tissue samples.

To encode the visual features of every WSI, the CNN features generated from the fine–tuned deep CNN network for prostate Gleason grading classification were extracted from the patches. The network architecture for pathology images presented in [17] was fine–tuned to classify five Gleason scores (6–10) instead of high vs. low cancer grading. In the end, 1024 dimensional feature vectors from the layer previous to the class probability output were extracted from each patch with the trained network.

Let S_a, S_b be the sets of selected RGB patches from two WSI at 40$\times$ resolution, in our setup $|S_a| = |S_b| = 2000$. Let $f(p) \in \mathbb{R}^{1024}$ be the function that takes a patch as input and computes the forward pass through the deep learning network up to the previous–to–last layer. For two patches $p_k \in S_a, p_l \in S_b$ we have $v^k = f(p_k)$ and $v^l = f(p_l)$, as the two CNN patch codes (or embeddings). The similarity between two patches is computed using the cosine similarity:

$$sim_{CNN}(v^k, v^l) = \frac{\sum_{i=1}^{1024} v_i^k v_i^l}{\sqrt{\sum_{i=1}^{1024} v_i^k}\sqrt{\sum_{i=1}^{1024} v_i^l}}$$

The visual similarity between the two slides is calculated adding all the similarities of the individual patches from each WSI:

$$sim_{\mathcal{V}}(S_a, S_b) = \sum_{k=1}^{2000}\sum_{l=1}^{2000} sim_{CNN}(v^k, v^l)$$

The cosine similarity is then computed between the vectors of a test query image and the vectors corresponding to each of the training WSIs. This results in a 2000×2000 similarity matrix for each pair of cases, which is added up to obtain a final visual similarity score.

2.3 Pathology Report Representation

Pathology reports contain information not only from the tissue samples but also from the surgical procedure performed to remove the tissue. This means that information not present in the histopathology images, such as tumor invasion to other body parts, is reported as well. Five criteria of diagnostic relevance for PRAD cases selected by a pathologist in addition to the Gleason score were extracted manually from the pathology reports. The selected criteria include the TNM classification of malignant tumors, with T (0–4) corresponding to the size of the tumor and invasion to nearby tissue and N (0–1) was marked as positive if lymph nodes were involved. Additionally, if the case showed angiolymphatic invasion of the tumor, perineural invasion or if the seminal vesicles were involved then each of these criteria was represented as 1, or 0 if absent. In cases with missing data, the lowest score was given to the corresponding criteria as their absence from the report could have signaled that it was not present during the interpretation. In the experiments, the Gleason score was excluded from the input criteria for the retrieval system.

Extracting the data from the reports automatically is not straightforward, as many regular expressions need to be formulated. For example, it is common to encounter the same grading written as *Gleason Score: 9, Primary pattern: 5, Secondary pattern: 4, score = 5 + 4, ...* This restricts the use of bag of words models because the pathology reports are not standardized. A more general approach was implemented to make use of unsupervised distributed models for embedding text content. We propose the representation of the text content from each report, embeddeding an n–dimensional space using an unsupervised distribution to a paragraph vector model of doc2vec [18]. Doc2vec is a suitable model for variable–length documents, as is the case of the pathology reports in the data set that were embedded into a 100 dimensional space. The text similarity was computed with the cosine similarity between the case embeddings and the similarity to the query cases was ranked according to this score. The proposed strategy can also be used for different types of tissue and different pathologies.

2.4 Multimodal Fusion

Let R_v, R_t, be the ranking for each query case, sorting the visual and text similarities. The generated late multimodal fusion rank R ranks the most relevant cases for the query by weighting the visual and textual similarities:

$$R = (1 - \alpha)R_v + \alpha R_t$$

In Fig. 2 a flowchart of the full approach is shown.

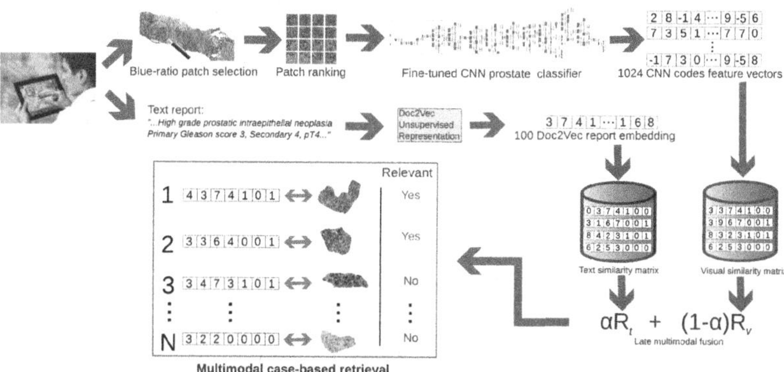

Fig. 2. Flowchart of the full multimodal approach. The pathology reports are embedded using doc2vec. The WSIs are represented as CNN–based features from automatically selected patches. A late fusion is performed between the similarity scores from both queries, obtaining the final multimodal ranking.

3 Experimental Results

The four retrieval methods for pathology cases presented in this paper were tested and compared. A retrieved case was considered relevant if the Gleason score from the case matched the query. To evalute the results, retrieval metrics from the NIST (US National Institute of Standards and Technology) evaluation procedures used in the Text Retrieval Conference (TREC) [19] were considered. The following five evaluation metrics were selected: mean average precision (MAP), geometric mean average precision (GM-MAP), binary preference (bpref), precision after 10 cases retrieved (P10) and precision after 30 cases retrieved (P30). The performance of each method is shown in Fig. 3.

The method *WS_CNN_Codes* used only visual features obtained from a fine–tuned CNN for Gleason grading classification, with 2000 selected patches at a 40× resolution per WSI. The model was trained using the Caffe framework and took 15 h to train with 2 NVIDIA Tesla K80 GPUs.

For text representation we tested two approaches, the first (*RepCateg*) computed a ranking based on the similarity of the report categories manually extracted from the pathologist reports, without including the Gleason score. The second text approach (*Rep2Vec*) was based on the unsupervised distributed representation of doc2vec [18]. Including or exculding information from the report regarding the Gleason grading was unsupervised. The gensim library was used with the default parameters and a total vocabulary of 3730 words, obtaining 100 dimensional vectors for each report. The ranking was generated using the cosine similarity between the doc2vec report representation.

The proposed multimodal approach (*Multimodal*) retrieved similar histopathology cases fusing the ranking generated by the deep CNN representation of the WSIs and the ranking from the embedded pathology report text using doc2vec. 10 values of α were explored in the range of $[0, 1]$. The best scores were obtained by the multimodal approach with $\alpha = 0.3$.

Method	*MAP*	*GM-MAP*	*bpref*	*P10*	*P30*
WS_CNN_Codes	0.5113	0.3921	0.4706	0.4500	0.4609
RepCateg	0.3522	0.3180	0.2759	0.3412	0.3399
Rep2Vec	0.4092	0.3561	0.3116	0.4913	0.3775
Multimodal	**0.5404**	**0.4196**	**0.4890**	**0.5217**	**0.4884**

(a) Evaluation results of four tested case–based retrieval approaches.

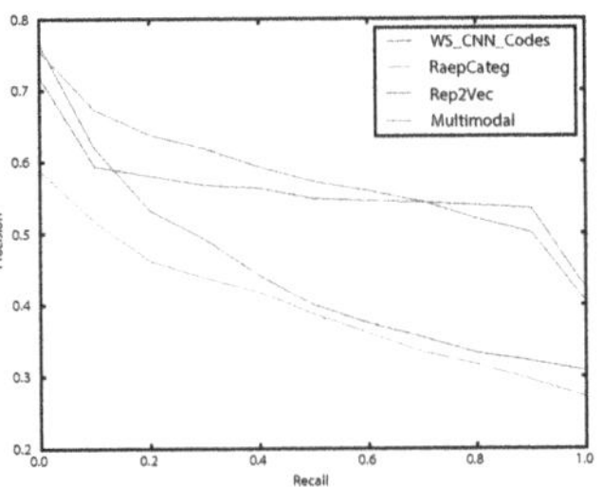

(b) Interpolated PR graph.

Fig. 3. Results from the text, visual and multimodal retrieval approaches.

4 Discussions

A multimodal case–based retrieval approach for histopathology cases based on visual features obtained with deep learning is presented in this paper with an automatic description of pathology reports. The main contributions are:

- This is the first multimodal histopathology strategy fusing visual features from WSIs and text embeddings of pathology reports, resulting in a novel case–based retrieval system.
- The method uses visual deep learning features for retrieval, representing WSIs, generated with a CNN trained to classify cancer gradings.
- The visual CNN model was trained with weakly annotated data (global Gleason scores from WSIs, without any manual annotations), and the free–form text embeddings obtained with an unsupervised approach.

The retrieval methods were trained, evaluated and compared on a publicly available test set. The visual–only approach (*WS CNN codes*) had better scores than both of the two text–only approaches: *RepCateg*, using 5 report criteria manually extracted and *Rep2Vec*, an unsupervised report to vector representation. This could be the result of training the visual representation of the cases with the 5 Gleason scores classes used to evaluate the relevance of the retrieved cases. Moreover, there is an intensive similarity computation among the CNN featires of the query case versus the remaining cases in the data set. When comparing both text–only approaches, embedding full–text reports to a vector, *Rep2Vec*, resulted in higher retrieval scores than *RepCateg*. *Rep2Vec* was able to better mimic the defined relevance of the retrieved cases, mainly because the selected criteria by a pathologist in the reports are only indirectly linked to the Gleason score. These criteria are focused on the surrounding organs and metastasic events which can be considered for another relevance measure of the cases.

The methods were trained and tested with images from several scanners and with no staining normalization. Adding such a normalization can improve performance. The TCGA data and the manual categories extracted from the reports are available for a fully reproducible setup of the proposed strategy. The multimodal fusion tested in this paper is simple as this is the very first example of retrieval fusing real medical reports and WSIs. More advanced fusion techniques can be implemented in a straightforward manner.

Most of the computations can be performed offline and a full case query can be performed in less than 8 s once the patches are extracted. The unsupervised retrieval system strategy was successful in obtaining cases with the same cancer grading even if these scores were not explicitly used in the text representations. The proposed retrieval system could be implemented, with minor modifications, for other organs and diseases. The task of assigning cancer gradings is strongly subjective. The cases retrieved could be better exploited to harmonize pathology case assessment and as a valuable resource for pathologists in training without depending on expensive and time consuming manual annotations.

Acknowledgments. This work was partially supported by the Eurostars project E! 9653 SLDESUTO-BOX. The authors would like to thank pathologist Lis Vázquez for her counsel regarding the handling of the pathology reports.

References

1. Müller, H., Michoux, N., Bandon, D., Geissbuhler, A.: A review of content-based image retrieval systems in medicine-clinical benefits and future directions. Int. J. Med. Inform. **73**(1), 1–23 (2004)
2. Begum, S., Ahmed, M.U., Funk, P., Xiong, N., Folke, M.: Case-based reasoning systems in the health sciences: a survey of recent trends and developments. IEEE Trans. Syst. Man Cybern. **41**(4), 421–434 (2011)
3. Welter, P., Deserno, T.M., Fischer, B., Günther, R.W., Spreckelsen, C.: Towards case-based medical learning in radiological decision making using content-based image retrieval. BMC Med. Inform. Decis. Making **11**, 68 (2011)

4. Jiménez-del-Toro, O.A., Hanbury, A., Langs, G., Foncubierta-Rodríguez, A., Müller, H.: Overview of the VISCERAL retrieval benchmark 2015. In: Müller, H., Jimenez del Toro, O.A., Hanbury, A., Langs, G., Foncubierta Rodriguez, A. (eds.) MRMD 2015. LNCS, vol. 9059, pp. 115–123. Springer, Cham (2015). doi:10.1007/978-3-319-24471-6_10
5. Caicedo, J.C., Vanegas, J.A., Páez, F., González, F.A.: Histology image search using multimodal fusion. J. Biomed. Inform. **51**, 114–128 (2014)
6. Zhang, X., Liu, W., Dundar, M., Badve, S., Zhang, S.: Towards large-scale histopathological image analysis: hashing-based image retrieval. IEEE Trans. Med. Imaging **34**(2), 496–506 (2015)
7. Kwak, J.T., Hewitt, S.M., Kajdacsy-Balla, A.A., Sinha, S., Bhargava, R.: Automated prostate tissue referencing for cancer detection and diagnosis. BMC Bioinform. **17**(1), 227 (2016)
8. Weinstein, R.S., Graham, A.R., Richter, L.C., Barker, G.P., Krupinski, E.A., Lopez, A.M., Erps, K.A., Bhattacharyya, A.K., Yagi, Y., Gilbertson, J.R.: Overview of telepathology, virtual microscopy, and whole slide imaging: prospects for the future. Hum. Pathol. **40**(8), 1057–1069 (2009)
9. Doyle, S., Hwang, M., Naik, S., Feldman, M., Tomaszeweski, J., Madabhushi, A.: Using manifold learning for content-based image retrieval of prostate histopathology. In: MICCAI 2007 Workshop on Content-based Image Retrieval for Biomedical Image Archives: Achievements, Problems, and Prospects, pp. 53–62. Citeseer (2007)
10. Krizhevsky, A., Hinton, G.E.: Using very deep autoencoders for content-based image retrieval. In: ESANN (2011)
11. Wu, P., Hoi, S.C., Xia, H., Zhao, P., Wang, D., Miao, C.: Online multimodal deep similarity learning with application to image retrieval. In: Proceedings of the 21st ACM International Conference on Multimedia, pp. 153–162. ACM (2013)
12. Wan, J., Wang, D., Hoi, S.C.H., Wu, P., Zhu, J., Zhang, Y., Li, J.: Deep learning for content-based image retrieval: a comprehensive study. In: Proceedings of the 22nd ACM International Conference on Multimedia, pp. 157–166. ACM (2014)
13. Gutman, D.A., Cobb, J., Somanna, D., Park, Y., Wang, F., Kurc, T., Saltz, J.H., Brat, D.J., Cooper, L.A.D., Kong, J.: Cancer digital slide archive: an informatics resource to support integrated in silico analysis of TCGA pathology data. J. Am. Med. Inform. Assoc. **20**(6), 1091–1098 (2013)
14. Ferlay, J., Soerjomataram, I., Dikshit, R., Eser, S., Mathers, C., Rebelo, M., Parkin, D.M., Forman, D., Bray, F.: Cancer incidence and mortality worldwide: sources, methods and major patterns in GLOBOCAN 2012. Int. J. Cancer **136**(5), E359–E386 (2015)
15. Humphrey, P.A.: Gleason grading and prognostic factors in carcinoma of the prostate. Mod. Pathol. **17**(3), 292–306 (2004)
16. LeCun, Y., Bengio, Y., Hinton, G.: Deep learning. Nature **521**(7553), 436–444 (2015)
17. Jimenez-del-Toro, O., Atzori, M., Otálora, S., Andersson, M., Eurén, K., Hedlund, M., Rönnquist, P., Müller, H.: Convolutional neural networks for an automatic classification of prostate tissue slides with high-grade gleason score. In: SPIE Medical Imaging. International Society for Optics and Photonics (2017)

18. Le, Q.V., Mikolov, T.: Distributed representations of sentences and documents. In: ICML, vol. 14, pp. 1188–1196 (2014)
19. Voorhees, E.M., Ellis, A. (eds.): Proceedings of The Twenty-Fourth Text REtrieval Conference, TREC 2015, Gaithersburg, Maryland, USA, 17–20 November 2015, vol. Special Publication 500–319. National Institute of Standards and Technology (NIST) (2015)

Sparse Representation Using Block Decomposition for Characterization of Imaging Patterns

Keni Zheng and Sokratis Makrogiannis(✉)

Mathematical Sciences Department, Delaware State University, Dover, DE 19901-2277, USA
smakrogiannis@desu.edu

Abstract. In this work we introduce sparse representation techniques for classification of high-dimensional imaging patterns into healthy and diseased states. We also propose a spatial block decomposition methodology that is used for training an ensemble of classifiers to address irregularities of the approximation problem. We first apply this framework to classification of bone radiography images for osteoporosis diagnosis. The second application domain is separation of breast lesions into benign and malignant. These are challenging classification problems because the imaging patterns are typically characterized by high Bayes error rate in the original space. To evaluate the classification performance we use cross-validation techniques. We also compare our sparse-based classification with state-of-the-art texture-based classification techniques. Our results indicate that decomposition into patches addresses difficulties caused by ill-posedness and improves original sparse classification.

1 Introduction

In the recent years, the development of accurate and reproducible computer-aided methods for timely diagnosis and prognosis of diseases has gained significant interest [2,10]. These techniques have the potential to have a significant impact on public health [7]. Early prediction can reduce the mortality rate from lethal diseases. In this paper, we introduce a system to separate healthy from diseased subjects using a block-based technique for sparse representation and classification. We test the predictive capability of our system for osteoporosis diagnosis and breast lesion characterization.

Osteoporosis is an age-related systemic bone skeletal disorder characterized by low bone mass and bone structure deterioration that results in increased

S. Makrogiannis—This research was supported by the National Institute of General Medical Sciences of the National Institutes of Health (NIH) under Award Number SC3GM113754 and by Intramural Research Program of NIA, NIH (Contract Number HHSN271201600204P). We also acknowledge the support by CREOSA of Delaware State University funded by NSF CREST-8763.

© Springer International Publishing AG 2017
G. Wu et al. (Eds.): Patch-MI 2017, LNCS 10530, pp. 158–166, 2017.
DOI: 10.1007/978-3-319-67434-6_18

bone fragility and higher fracture risk [2]. Therefore, early diagnosis can effectively predict fracture risk and prevent the disease. Furthermore, breast cancer is one of the leading causes of death among women [7]. If the breast cancer can be diagnosed early, when it is small and has not spread, it can be treated successfully. Hence early detection and characterization of breast lesions is very important for preventing deaths. Mammograms can help to detect and diagnose breast cancer at an early stage. Automated diagnosis in both applications is very challenging since scans of healthy and diseased subjects show little or no visual differences, and their density histograms have significant overlap.

Sparse representation methods have been applied to a wide range of fields including coding, feature extraction and classification, superresolution, and regularization of inverse problems [8, 11–13]. In addition, sparse representation may provide insight into significant patterns that form object category prototypes. Sparse representation techniques describe a vector sample by sparse linear combinations of atoms from an overcomplete dictionary of prototypes. If these representations are sparse enough, then the representations reveal characteristic imaging patterns of disease and can be used for object recognition and classification. The authors in [11] proposed the sparse representation classification (SRC) method to recognize 2,414 frontal-face images of 38 individuals of Yale B Database and over 4,000 frontal images for 126 individuals of AR Database. The recognition rates were above 90% for both databases. The SRC approach with dictionary learning has also been applied to classification of pulmonary patterns of diffuse lung diseases [13]. 1161 volumes of interest were used for classification and this method yielded high class separation. Other approaches such as WGSR and Modular SRC methods [12] propose to partition the image into blocks to address the occurrence of occlusions in face recognition.

In this work, we introduce our block decomposition-based classification method that uses sparse representations of imaging patterns. This technique helps to overcome numerical optimization difficulties such as convergence to infeasible solutions. In addition, the introduction of a classifier ensemble approach aims to improve classification accuracy. We validated the proposed technique for separation of healthy from osteoporotic subjects femur bone radiographs with an accuracy of 96.6% and separation of benign from malignant lesions in mammograms with accuracy of 82.2%. We also performed comparisons with the traditional SRC technique and observed improvements of 12.1% in bone characterization and 17.8% in breast lesion characterization. Additional cross-validation experiments indicate that our patch-based sparse analysis method outperforms texture-based state-of-the-art classifiers. Therefore, this technique may be applicable to computer-aided diagnosis.

2 Methods

2.1 Sparse Representation and Classification

Sparse Representation techniques construct a dictionary from labeled training samples to calculate a linear representation of a test sample. This representation can be used to make a decision for the class of the test sample. Assuming that a dataset has k distinct classes, s samples, and for the ith class there are s_i samples, so that $s = \sum_i s_i$, we define a dictionary matrix M from the training set as $M = [v_{1,1}, v_{1,2}, ..., v_{k,s_k}]$, where $M \in \mathbb{R}^{l \times s}$, and $v_{i,h}$ is a column vector for the hth sample from ith class. In image classification applications, a $p \times q$ grayscale image forms a vector $v \in \mathbb{R}^l$, $l = p \times q$ using lexicographical ordering.

A new test sample $y \in \mathbb{R}^l$, can be represented by a linear combination of samples $y = \sum_{i=1}^{k} \beta_{i,1} v_{i,1} + \beta_{i,2} v_{i,2} + \cdots + \beta_{i,s_i} v_{i,s_i}$, where $\beta_{i,h} \in \mathbb{R}$ are scalar coefficients. Hence, the test sample y can be rewritten as:

$$y = Mx_0 \in \mathbb{R}^l. \tag{1}$$

where x_0 is a sparse solution. If there are sufficient training samples, the components of x_0 are equal to zero except for the components corresponding to the ith class. Then $x_0 = [0, 0, ..., \beta_{i,1}, \beta_{i,2}, ..., \beta_{i,s_i}, 0, 0, ..., 0]^T \in \mathbb{R}^s$.

In [6], it was proved that whenever $y = Mx$ for some x, if there are less than $l/2$ nonzero entries in x, x is the unique sparse solution: $\widehat{x}_0 = x$. Finding the sparse solution of an underdetermined system of linear equations is an NP-hard problem [1]. The authors in [3–5] supported that if the solution x_0 is sparse enough, it is equal to the solution $\widehat{x}$ of the l^1-minimization problem:

$$(l^1): \quad \widehat{x} = \arg\min ||x||_1 \quad s.t. \quad Mx = y. \tag{2}$$

In sparse representation classification we define a characteristic function $\delta_i : \mathbb{R}^s \rightarrow \mathbb{R}^s$ that has nonzero entries, only if x is associated with class i. Then the function $\widehat{y}_i = M\delta_i(\widehat{x})$, represents the given sample y using components from class i only. To classify y, we minimize the residual between y and $\widehat{y}_i$ [11]: $\omega_i = \arg\min_i r_i(y) \doteq \arg\min_i ||y - M\delta_i(\widehat{x})||_2$.

We utilize the interior point solver method to solve the problem in (2), formulated as a linear programming (LP) problem. An LP problem is a constrained optimization problem that seeks the minimizer of a linear objective function subject to linear constraints [9].

2.2 Block-Based Sparse Representation for Classification

Spatial Decomposition into Blocks. The images that we use for lesion characterization are subject to intra-class variability, that cause the samples to depart from the true class prototype. Furthermore, the high dimensionality of the feature space complicates the optimization procedure and may lead to infeasible solutions. We propose a block-based sparse representation classifier to overcome these problems.

Figure 1 outlines the main steps of our approach. We partition each training image into non-overlapping blocks with size $m \times n$ each. Therefore, each image is represented as $I = [B^1, B^2, ..., B^{NB}]$, where NB is the number of image blocks. The dictionary D_j, where $j = 1, 2, ..., NB$ is corresponding to the same position of the patch for each image. The dictionary D^j for the block B^j can be written as follows for all s images:

$$D^j = [bv^j_{1,1}, bv^j_{1,2}, \ldots, bv^j_{k,s_k}], \tag{3}$$

where $bv^j_{i,h}$ is column block vector for the hth sample, ith class, jth block B^j.

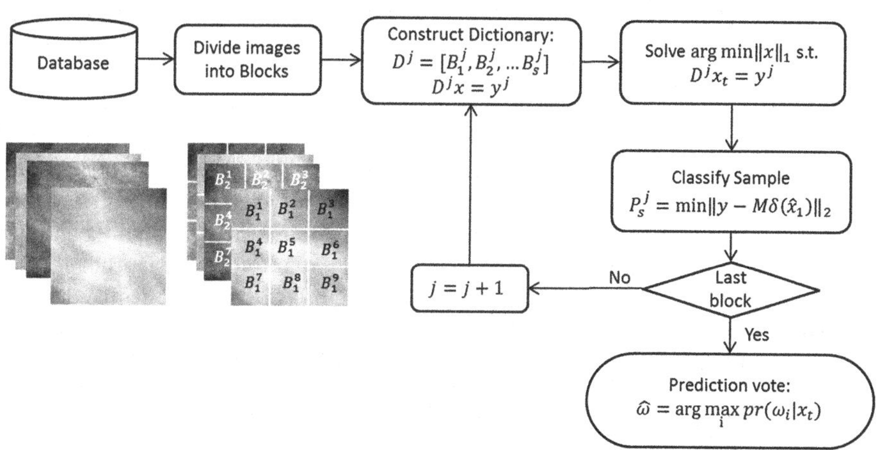

Fig. 1. Main stages of the block-based sparse representation-based classifier.

Block-Based Classification. We propose to solve an ensemble of sparse representation classification problems to classify each test sample. Given a test sample y^j obtained from the jth block, we approximate the solution x^j by linear programming:

$$\hat{x}^j = \arg\min ||x^j||_1, \quad \text{subject to,} \quad D^j x = y^j, \tag{4}$$

where $j = 1, 2, ..., NB$. We then assign the test sample y^j to the class that produces the minimum approximation error as in SRC. So y^j is classified into ω^j_i, where $i = 1, \ldots, k$ is the class index.

Voting Decision Function. The class decision for each image is completed by voting over the ensemble of NB block-based classifiers. The predicted class label $\hat{\omega}$ is given by

$$\hat{\omega} = \arg\max_i pr(\omega_i|\hat{x}), \tag{5}$$

where $\hat{x}$ is the composite extracted feature from the test sample given by the solution of (4), and $pr(\omega_i|\hat{x}) = \sum_j^{NB} n_{\omega^j_i}/NB$ is the likelihood for classifying $\hat{x}$ into class ω_i, and $n_{\omega^j_i}$ is an indicator function such that $n_{\omega^j_i} = 1$, only if the j-th classifier made the decision ω_i, otherwise it is 0.

3 Results and Discussion

Here we describe the main experiments that we performed to validate the classification performance of our system. The application domain is computer-aided disease diagnosis. We concentrate on bone characterization and breast lesion characterization. In both applications there is significant overlap between the intensity distributions of healthy and diseased subjects.

We measured the classification performance of our block-based sparse representation approach by calculating the true positive rate (TPR), true negative rate (TNR), classification accuracy (ACC), and area under the ROC curve (AUC) in leave-one-out cross-validation experiments. We also performed the same classification experiments for the conventional SRC. Finally, we employed the texture-based classification techniques described in [14] for further comparisons. We computed texture features based on wavelet decomposition, discrete Fourier and Cosine transforms, fractal dimension, statistical co-occurrence indices, and structural texture descriptors. Next, we employed feature selection methods (FSM) using a correlation-based functional criterion optimized using a best-first search strategy (CFS-BF), or genetic algorithm optimization (CFS-GA). In the classification stage we employed Naive Bayes (NB), Bayes Network (BN), Random Forests (RF), and Bagging models for diagnosis.

In our first experiment we aimed to separate healthy from osteoporotic subjects. We used the TCB challenge dataset, which includes annotated images of 58 healthy and 58 osteoporotic subjects that display a region of interest with size 400×400 pixels in the trabecular bone. The TCB challenge data is publicly available online from http://www.univ-orleans.fr/i3mto/data. We employed the SRC method to classify the whole ROIs after undersampling by variable factors to reduce the occurrence of numerical difficulties such as infeasible solutions mainly caused by linearly dependent vectors that yielded different classes. In the first two rows in Table 1 we display results from the top performing experiments yielding a classification accuracy of 84.5% for resampling of 1/20 corresponding to a dimensionality of 400 in the feature domain. Higher degree of downsampling produces shorter and more numerically tractable feature dimensionality, but it also diffuses the textural information.

Next, we validated the performance of the proposed approach that operates on image patches. We varied the block sizes from 100×100 pixels to 5×5 pixels to investigate the effect of this variable on classification performance. We display our cross-validation results in Table 1. The best performing classification of 96.6% was achieved for a block size of 8×8 pixels that resulted in 2500 classifiers. This implies a 12.1% improvement over the traditional SRC approach. These results suggest that the block-based approach finds more sparse solutions and improves the classifier performance.

The TCB data set is very difficult to classify therefore the solution obtained by the original SRC technique may not always be sparse. To obtain a sparse solution we need to construct dictionary matrices with linearly independent vectors and to reduce the number of unknowns. The block-based analysis aims to render

Table 1. Classification performance for bone characterization using sparse representation. The block size in first two rows implies no block decomposition (as in original SRC).

Size of block	TPR (%)	TNR (%)	ACC (%)	AUC (%)
400 × 400 (undersamp. 1/4)	84.5	67.2	75.9	74.6
400 × 400 (undersamp. 1/20)	87.9	81.0	84.5	81.9
100 × 100	46.6	100	73.3	71.2
50 × 50	51.7	100	75.9	74.3
25 × 25	69.0	100	85.0	80.7
20 × 20	72.4	100	86.2	83.7
10 × 10	87.9	100	94.0	93.3
8 × 8	**93.1**	**100**	**96.6**	**96.9**
5 × 5	100	82.8	91.4	92.8

this inverse problem more numerically tractable by reducing the dimensionality of samples and by introducing an ensemble meta-algorithm for decision making.

In Table 2 we report the classification rates produced by texture-based classifiers in leave-one-out cross-validation experiments. We note that the top performance is achieved when using CFS-BF followed by classification by a Bayes network BN. The classification accuracy is 79.3% and the area under the curve is 81%. Both rates are lower than those produced by the proposed method. In our second experiment we validated the classification of suspicious breast lesions into benign and malignant classes. We obtained data from the public Mammographic Image Analysis Society (MIAS) database to test our method. The mammograms have a resolution of 200 micron pixel edge and have been clipped/padded so that

Table 2. Classification performance for bone characterization using texture-based classification techniques.

FSM	CL	TPR (%)	TNR (%)	ACC (%)	AUC (%)	Dimension
CFS-GA	NB	50.0	62.1	56.0	57.6	137
	BN	77.6	67.2	72.4	76.7	
	RF	65.5	60.3	62.9	65.0	
	Bagging	53.4	63.8	58.6	62.5	
CFS-BF	NB	72.4	60.3	66.4	71.6	6 (29, 129, 166, 561, 599, 636)
	BN	**82.8**	**75.9**	**79.3**	**81.0**	
	RF	74.1	69.0	71.6	76.2	
	Bagging	69.0	72.4	70.7	76.0	

every image is 1024 pixels × 1024 pixels. In this experiment we used the centroid and radius information for each lesion to determine a square ROI of the same size for each scan.

We then applied our block-based classification system and cross-validated its performance as in our first experiment. In Table 3 we report the results produced by use of ROI size equal to 64 × 64 pixels that resulted in 36 benign and 37 malignant lesions that contain the ROI. In this table the first row corresponds to the use of a single block that is equivalent to the traditional SRC method. Our system achieved a classification accuracy of 82.2% for block size of 16 × 16. We note an improvement of 17.8 % over the conventional SRC method indicating that the block decomposition yields more accurate representation of the test samples than SRC. The voting decision function contributes to reduction of potential prediction variance. Furthermore, in Table 4 we report the performance of texture-based classifiers. The highest classification accuracy of 76.6% is achieved using CFS-BF and Bayes Network. CFS-BF and RF classification yielded the top area under ROC curve at 79.2%. CFS-BF combined with RF or Bagging techniques produced the same TPR, TNR and ACC measurements. Overall, the proposed block-based sparse classifier outperforms texture-based classification.

Table 3. Classification performance for breast lesion characterization using sparse representation (ROI size: 64 × 64). The block size in first row implies no block decomposition (as in original SRC).

Size of block	TPR (%)	TNR (%)	ACC (%)	AUC (%)
64 × 64	56.8	72.2	64.4	64.0
32 × 32	56.8	88.9	72.6	73.5
16 × 16	**70.3**	**94.4**	**82.2**	**82.9**
8 × 8	62.2	94.4	78.1	76.3
4 × 4	67.6	55.6	61.6	58.9

Table 4. Classification performance for breast lesion characterization using texture-based classification techniques (ROI size: 60 × 60).

FSM	CL	TPR (%)	TNR (%)	ACC (%)	AUC (%)	Dimension
CFS-GA	NB	67.5	35.1	51.9	55.8	54
	BN	77.5	64.9	71.4	59.9	
	RF	70.0	59.5	64.9	63.9	
	Bagging	60.0	56.8	58.4	65.0	
CFS-BF	NB	77.5	45.9	62.3	70.6	4 (119, 143, 322, 397)
	BN	**77.5**	**75.7**	**76.6**	**71.0**	
	RF	75.0	73.0	74.0	**79.2**	
	Bagging	75.0	73.0	74.0	77.1	

4 Conclusion

We proposed a block-based sparse representation and classification approach. We validated the classification performance for two disease diagnostics applications; bone characterization in digital radiographs and breast lesion characterization in mammograms. We compared our results with the performance of the conventional SRC method and with various texture-based non-sparse classification techniques. The proposed method produced classification rates of 96.6% for bone characterization and 82.2% for breast lesion characterization. Our results indicate that the introduction of patch analysis yields more accurate solutions than the compared methods. The proposed system has the potential to contribute to identification of individuals with higher risk of disease and for early intervention.

References

1. Amaldi, E., Kann, V.: On the approximability of minimizing nonzero variables or unsatisfied relations in linear systems. Theoret. Comput. Sci. **209**(1), 237–260 (1998)
2. Bartl, R., Frisch, B.: Osteoporosis: Diagnosis, Prevention, Therapy. Springer Science & Business Media, Heidelberg (2009)
3. Candès, E.J., Romberg, J.K., Tao, T.: Stable signal recovery from incomplete and inaccurate measurements. Commun. Pure Appl. Math. **59**(8), 1207–1223 (2006)
4. Candès, E.J., Tao, T.: Near-optimal signal recovery from random projections: Universal encoding strategies? IEEE Trans. Inf. Theory **52**(12), 5406–5425 (2006)
5. Donoho, D.L.: For most large underdetermined systems of linear equations the minimal l1-norm solution is also the sparsest solution. Comm. Pure Appl. Math. **59**(6), 797–829 (2004)
6. Donoho, D.L., Elad, M.: Optimally sparse representation in general (nonorthogonal) dictionaries via l1 minimization. Proc. Nat. Acad. Sci. **100**(5), 2197–2202 (2003)
7. Ferlay, J., Héry, C., Autier, P., Sankaranarayanan, R.: Global burden of breast cancer. In: Li, C. (ed.) Breast Cancer Epidemiology, pp. 1–19. Springer, New York (2010). doi:10.1007/978-1-4419-0685-4_1
8. Qiao, L., Chen, S., Tan, X.: Sparsity preserving projections with applications to face recognition. Pattern Recogn. **43**(1), 331–341 (2010)
9. Robere, R.: Interior point methods and linear programming. Technical report, University of Toronto (2012)
10. Smith, R.A., Cokkinides, V., Eyre, H.J.: American cancer society guidelines for the early detection of cancer, 2003. CA Cancer J. Clin. **53**(1), 27–43 (2003)
11. Wright, J., Yang, A.Y., Ganesh, A., Sastry, S.S., Ma, Y.: Robust face recognition via sparse representation. IEEE Trans. Pattern Anal. Mach. Intell. **31**(2), 210–227 (2009)
12. Zhao, S.-H., Hu, Z.-P.: Occluded face recognition based on block-label and residual. Int. J. Artif. Intell. Tools **25**(03), 1650019 (2016)

13. Zhao, W., Xu, R., Hirano, Y., Tachibana, R., Kido, S.: A sparse representation based method to classify pulmonary patterns of diffuse lung diseases. Comput. Math. Methods Med. **2015**, 567932 (2015)
14. Zheng, K., Makrogiannis, S.: Bone texture characterization for osteoporosis diagnosis using digital radiography. In: 2016 38th Annual International Conference of the IEEE Engineering in Medicine and Biology Society (EMBC), pp. 1034–1037, August 2016

Author Index

Printed in the United States
By Bookmasters